UNDERSTANDING

AIDS

A CANADIAN STRATEGY

UNDERSTANDING

AIDS

A CANADIAN STRATEGY

Royal Society
of Canada

DAVID SPURGEON

KEY PORTER·BOOKS

Canadian Cataloguing in Publication Data

Spurgeon, David, 1925-
    Understanding AIDS

ISBN 1-55013-124-9

1. AIDS (Disease) — Social aspects — Canada.
I. Title.

RC607.A26S68 1988	362.1'969792	C88-094343-2

Key Porter Books Limited
70 The Esplanade
Toronto, Ontario
Canada M5E 1R2

Printed and Bound in Canada

88   89   90   91   92   6   5   4   3   2   1

Contents

Preface

This book was commissioned by the Royal Society of Canada and supported by it financially. It was written while members of the Society's expert committee were preparing the recently published study, *AIDS: A Perspective for Canadians.* By initiating and supporting a book aimed directly at the general reader, officials of the Society hope to gain a wider consideration of the ideas contained in this official report. They consider this essential because of the urgent need for all Canadians to understand the nature of the AIDS epidemic.

The book draws heavily on the Royal Society's report. That report was, in fact, my primary-source document, and I tried throughout to adhere to its spirit and intent. However, I also sought information from a variety of other authorities, not the least being those who spoke at a special symposium on AIDS at the annual meeting of the American Association for the Advancement of Science in Boston, Massachusetts, in February, 1988.

While writing the book I was also privileged to attend meetings of the Royal Society's panel of experts, and profited from their advice and assistance, as well as from the comments of some on the manuscript. I am particularly indebted to the project co-ordinator, Dr. Maung T. (Bertie) Aye, head of hematology at Ottawa General Hospital, for his advice, his close collaboration and his support. The author is, however, solely responsible for its contents.

Introduction

The acronym AIDS (for Acquired Immunodeficiency Syndrome) has, in a mere six years, become familiar to every Canadian. It is almost impossible to pick up a copy of a newspaper or magazine without seeing AIDS articles. AIDS items appear with the monotony of commercials on nightly televison newscasts. And AIDS books have begun to fill bookstores and libraries; the 1986 edition of *Books in Print* listed 84 publications on the subject, while a 1987 Canadian Public Health Association Report on AIDS/STD Education for Youth listed 77 films about AIDS and STD (sexually transmitted diseases), 80 books in English and 39 in French.

Why then publish yet another AIDS study?

One reason is that AIDS is a moving target: much still remains unknown about the disease and its possible impacts, and we need to keep up with the latest findings. Some of these findings are difficult for the general reader who finds little help in the apparently contradictory nature of many news reports, to evaluate. Access to the balanced and considered judgment of qualified observers is difficult. Many books expressing the opinions of individuals have been published, but few (if any in Canada) contain the consensus of a wide range of experts in relevant fields, as does this one. But a more compelling reason is that despite the flood of material already published, none yet seems to have grappled with the question: What are the overall implications of AIDS for Canadian society as a whole, and how best can we, as Canadians, meet the medical and social challenge the expected epidemic presents?

It was for this reason that the Royal Society of Canada undertook, in the summer of 1987, to set up a series of panels to review the most up-to-date, factual data available on AIDS and, in the light of this, to make recommendations in areas of pressing public concern. The idea was to look at AIDS not just as a medical problem — though medical and public-health aspects obviously are of major importance — but comprehensively, as a disease with unprecedented social, legal, ethical and economic ramifications.

A primary motivation for the study was to respond to the atmosphere of fear surrounding what has often been described as "a new plague." Members of the Royal Society of Canada realized that, as a result of this fear, and because of the way the disease is transmitted and the fact that no adequate treatment or cure is available, it could easily lead to the victimization and ostracization of a large and growing sector of Canadian society. Signs of this happening have already appeared: by late 1987, a teacher in Nova Scotia had been removed from his classroom because he was identified as an AIDS-virus carrier (he was later reinstated but almost immediately resigned to join a provincial panel on AIDS). A private school in Ontario instituted mandatory testing for the virus antibody among all its pupils and teachers, and another decided it would call for selective testing whenever it thought a risk existed. And compulsory AIDS tests for immigrants were being advocated in some quarters.

The implications of such actions for Canadian society — traditionally a humane, tolerant and caring one — are alarming. We have in this country what is widely recognized as one of the best health-care plans in the world. We are regarded abroad, especially in developing countries, as a refuge for the oppressed, wherein political and personal freedoms flourish. Yet the fear of AIDS is driving some Canadians to propose actions that could bring into question many of these assumptions. Here, as in other countries, the way in which we handle this distressing situation will be a test of our civilization.

There are also more practical considerations to confront. How will we as Canadians cope with this disease if it takes on the dimensions many are predicting for it? Without effective treatments, what shall we do with AIDS sufferers? How will they fit into our much-vaunted health-care system? Where, physically, will they be put? Into active treatment hospitals, which already suffer shortages of space, personnel, equipment and funds? Into special facilities, which again pose the question of segregation, and which in any case have yet to be funded and built? And how funded? How many such patients will we have to deal with, since current projections of the spread of the disease vary? Who will pay for all this and what effect will the new demands have on both government-run health-insurance plans and on private life and disability-insurance policies?

The AIDS epidemic is sure to have legal implications. What will these be? The attitudes born of fear may well affect AIDS sufferers in ways that will conflict with the Canadian Charter of Rights and Freedoms. The time to anticipate those ways is now, not when the problem is upon us. For example, what are the implications for the functioning of the Criminal Code, and for those already in prisons?

As readers will learn later in this book, public education is seen as a fundamentally important way to meet the AIDS problem. How will this education be carried out? By whom? And how much will it cost and who will pay for it? What are the special implications for the training of doctors, nurses and paramedical personnel? And how will these new demands be met?

Because much remains to be understood about the disease and ways to cope with it, increased research in both the medical and social sciences will become necessary. This will require increased funding. At a time when such research in Canada is badly under-funded compared with that in other developed countries, where will this money come from and how will it be administered?

Such are the kinds of question this book seeks to answer. It is not designed to frighten the reader with terrifying statistics and stories of personal agony (though it does include the latest figures on incidence in Canada, and a poignant personal case history). Its starting point is that we all now *know* AIDS is a fearsome disease that can affect all of us. Some believe it is a threat to the very fabric of our society. Others would prefer to ignore it and hope it will eventually somehow disappear, or that we will be saved from disaster by medical science. Whatever our perceptions of the threat of AIDS, this book seeks to pose the question, what can we *do* about it? Its aim is to provide, in a dispassionate way, the known facts — as well as what is not known and what is uncertain — together with the issues and arguments that will allow Canadians individually to answer this question in their own way. In doing so, it will also allow us to see how our society has already begun to react to the disease, what the implications of these actions are, and whether they seem an appropriate response.

To a degree, the Royal Society's findings are reassuring: they suggest that both the cumulative number of cases previously predicted to 1992 and the estimated number of persons now infected could be smaller than feared. Compared with other causes of death for males aged 25-44, AIDS ranked only tenth in 1985, following suicide, motor-vehicle accidents, coronary heart disease, stroke and cirrhosis. Yet such findings leave no cause for complacency: preliminary data for 1986 suggest AIDS has already moved up to fourth place. And if current epidemiological trends remain constant, deaths from AIDS could surpass those from coronary heart disease to make it the third leading cause of death for males in this age group — and by 1992 it could even become the primary cause.

Whatever happens, the cost to Canada will be high. These costs are estimated for the first time in this study. They show that by 1992, direct expenditures (i.e. treatment and prevention) could amount to 1.2-2.1 percent of the country's health-care expenditures; they were in 1987 about 0.3 percent. Indirect costs (the value of the loss to society when a person dies prematurely) run even higher — in 1987 from 0.3-0.6 percent of the country's gross domestic product.

In the face of such a challenge as AIDS, some of the recommendations made by the Royal Society are bound to be controversial, for example the proposal that condoms be made available by correctional institutions for their inmates to help prevent the spread of the AIDS virus. Or the recommendation that free needles and syringes, and facilities for decontaminating needles, be made available to drug users.

The contentious question of testing to see whether an individual has been infected by the AIDS virus is explored in detail, and the examination reveals much not generally known about the uncertainty of test results. The implications of testing for discrimination of various kinds, and the need to safeguard confidentiality of test results, are thoroughly explored, and proposals calling for mandatory testing of all hospital patients, of immigrants and of students and teachers and other school employees, are rejected outright. Similarly, changes are called for in reporting laws to provide that the reporting of AIDS cases or of infection by the AIDS virus should not identify the person.

Recommendations are made for the improvement of social benefits for people with AIDS and their families — including the provision of subsidized housing for those whose condition causes housing problems, and the compensation of those infected with the AIDS virus through blood transfusions. And finally, proposals are put forward for the organization of medical care for AIDS patients, and for the better functioning of research into the disease itself.

Writing in *Issues in Science and Technology* (Winter, 1986), June E. Osborn, dean of the University of Michigan's School of Public Health, said of AIDS: "For the first time in modern history a worldwide epidemic of an entirely novel, lethal viral disease has begun under close scientific scrutiny." But she added: "Only some of the keys to its solution lie in the realm of biomedical science . . . . From the outset it has been impossible to deal with AIDS only in the context of the natural sciences because of the intimate admixture of issues involving sociology, psychology, ethics and the law."

This book sets forth some of the responses of a number of Canadian leaders from these fields to the unique challenge of AIDS. Their recommendations (listed at the end of the book) constitute the first attempt in Canada to draw up a comprehensive plan of action with which Canadian society can meet this challenge. Although, as might be expected, members of the Royal Society of Canada's panel of experts disagreed about specific points during their discussions, it is remarkable that consensus was reached not only on the main thrust of their report, but on every recommendation proposed.

The book is meant to be read by the general public. For the most part it is non-technical, and where scientific terms or concepts are described, they are explained in lay language. The first chapter, which tells what is known about the origin and spread of the AIDS virus, "The Trojan Horse Caper," and part of Chapter Three, "The Testing Dilemma," are the most scientifically detailed. Chapter One could be skipped by those already familiar with this material or those not desiring such detail, or it could be referred to later. It can serve, however, as a source of scientifically accurate information about the disease — something not always available in popular material about AIDS. The technical part of Chapter Three is likewise not essential for the understanding of the major issues in the testing dilemma. Those who wish to get to the heart of the social problems AIDS poses might therefore begin with Chapter Two: "AIDS in Perspective."

The kinds of social, ethical and legal problems AIDS poses are described in Chapter Four: "Could AIDS Transform Canadian

Society?'' illustrated by a case history. Chapter Five: ''The Price to Pay,'' estimates the cost of AIDS to Canada so far and in the future and makes proposals for organization of medical care for persons with AIDS. Chapter Six: ''What Can Be Done?'' discusses the main hope for stemming the AIDS epidemic — education. And Chapter Seven: ''The Future,'' makes some proposals not only for new directions for AIDS research, but for what the ordinary Canadian can do to help meet the AIDS challenge.

CHAPTER ONE

The Trojan Horse Caper

During the 1940s, a strange epidemic occurred among sheep imported into Iceland from Germany. The sheep, previously healthy, began suffering from shortness of breath, appeared to become partly paralyzed and then gradually and slowly wasted away and died.

An Icelandic physician, Bjorn Sigurdsson, became interested and in 1958 published an article in a British medical journal showing that there were actually two diseases involved. He showed further that they were caused by two different viruses, which he named *visna* (wasting) and *maedi* (shortness of breath), after the Icelandic names for the symptoms they caused. And because the symptoms came on slowly, he introduced the term lentivirus, or slow infection, to characterize the family of virus to which they belong.

We now know that the virus that causes AIDS also belongs to this family: all three are subfamilies of a family called retroviruses. A retrovirus literally means a "backward virus" because it works "in reverse" compared to body cells and other viruses. Ordinary viruses are simply extremely small packets of genetic material surrounded by a protein coat. The genetic material in viruses is usually deoxyribonucleic acid, or DNA, as it is in our body cells. In body cells, DNA is chemically coded into messages called genes. It is these messages that direct the making of protein in forms that determine all the characteristics of the individual. This is normally done through the medium of "messenger RNA": the genetic message is transferred from DNA by means of an RNA template. Retroviruses reverse this process with the help of an enzyme called reverse transcriptase: this enzyme allows the genetic messages of a virus made of RNA to be transferred to DNA.

Interestingly, the subfamilies of the retroviruses include not only lentiviruses such as *visna* and *maedi* and the AIDS virus, but also oncoviruses, which cause cancers in animals, birds and reptiles, and man. Thus the Icelandic doctor's findings with sheep set the stage for the discovery of diseases that work slowly and insidiously in man — discoveries that have only just begun to lead researchers into what one day could help medical scientists unravel that greatest of medical mysteries, the mechanism of cancer.

The silent intruders
The most interesting aspect of the lentiviruses is what microbiologist Ashley T. Haase of the University of Minnesota called in an article in the British journal *Nature* their "immunologically silent nature." Once a lentivirus manages to infect a cell, it does its dirty work unnoticed by the body's immune system — the body's defence mechanisms. These mechanisms use white blood cells and antibodies to destroy or neutralize foreign invaders when they come across them in the body. Antibodies are protein molecules produced by the body when foreign invaders, such as viruses or bacteria, enter the bloodstream. Each individual type of antibody is designed specifically to react with a particular invader, so as to protect the body against it. The lentiviruses have the ability to invade a body cell and take over its genetic mechanism, so that instead of doing its usual work the cell is virtually turned into a virus factory, producing thousands of copies of the virus, which assemble at the cell's surface. Yet until this stage of active assembly, the virus hides out in the cell; it sits silently inside, undetectable because it has ceased to exist in its original form and has actually become part of the cell.

A similar immunologically silent mechanism explains how the lentivirus can circulate and spread through the bloodstream, cerebrospinal fluid and the other bodily fluids containing bodily defence cells such as antibodies — and even penetrate the so-called blood-brain barrier directly into the brain. To do this, it hides out like a sort of invisible hitchhiker in one of the defensive cells that move constantly through the body, and that mobile cell takes it, unobserved, to other sites, which it then infects. Because of the analogy to the Greek myth, this trick of the lentivirus has been dubbed the "Trojan horse mechanism." It is an artful and effective way in which lentiviruses avoid discovery and destruction by their enemies. Such subterfuges also provide the reason why the AIDS virus is so difficult to defeat medically.

Where did the AIDS virus come from?
The AIDS virus is truly a new phenomenon to medical science in many respects. Its origin is unknown, though some evidence suggests the human AIDS virus had a common ancestor with the virus found in several African monkeys, and that it somehow was transferred to humans, thus crossing the "species barrier." No one knows how this could have happened. Nor is it known where the disease first arose. Evidence has been found of AIDS-like diseases in Africa in the late 1970s, but there is also evidence that it appeared in the United States and Haiti about the same time. In a recent case, the AIDS virus was found in preserved body specimens of an American teenager who died from a mysterious disease in 1969. In "AIDS; An International Perspective," in the February 5, 1988 issue of the Americal journal *Science*, Dr. Peter Piot of Belgium's Institute of Tropical Medicine and colleagues noted that the first recognition and report of AIDS occurred in 1981 when antibody to the AIDS virus was found in blood that had been stored in Zaire in 1959. But they add: "However, similar studies on stored blood have not been reported from Europe or North America, and no conclusions can be drawn as to the origin of AIDS." Dr. Jonathan Mann, director of the World Health Organization's AIDS program has written: "The complete history of AIDS will probably remain a mystery."

Electron microscopy is gradually revealing what the virus looks like. For an organism that can do so much damage, it is amazingly small: a cube made up of a billion viruses packed together would just be visible to the naked eye. Its shape resembles a soccer ball. The outer layer is the protein coat, while the RNA core is believed to be curled into the shape of a hollow cone with a dimpled large end like that of a champagne bottle.

The virus can enter only certain types of cells in the human body: those that have receptors on their surfaces to which the virus can bind. These receptors are normal appendages of the cells, used for their own purposes, but for the AIDS virus they provide a convenient attachment point.

Most important from the point of view of the AIDS virus are the receptors on the surface of a type of white blood cell called T4 cells. These cells are a vital part of the body's protection against disease: they orchestrate the entire immune system with instructions that co-ordinate its fight against invaders. After attaching themselves to the receptors on T4 cells, the AIDS virus enters the cells either through an invagination of the cell membrane or by fusing with the membrane.

How the virus works
Once inside, the virus disintegrates, releasing its RNA and the reverse transcriptase enzyme. It is at this point that the real infection takes place. The reverse transcriptase copies the viral RNA and translates it into DNA. This viral DNA then enters the cell's nucleus and becomes incorporated with the cell's own DNA. The viral DNA is now a permanent part of the infected person's cell, and the virus as it was when it entered the cell no longer exists. Because the virus's and the cell's genetic material have become virtually one and the same, the human cell has now become a sort of progenitor virus, "pro-virus," ready at any time to duplicate the original virus.

When the pro-virus receives a signal from other parts of the immune system — alerting it perhaps to the arrival of another infectious agent, or antigen — the cell of the infected person suddenly springs into action and starts producing virus particles. These particles push through the cell wall, acquiring portions of it as they do so, and finally breaking free as complete viruses. Once outside the cell, these new viruses are free to spread within the body, just as their progenitor was, and they go on to infect not just other T4 cells but different kinds of cells such as those in the brain. In a final coup, as they leave the body cells that have produced them, the new viruses kill them, thus further disabling the immune system. Because of its effects on this system, the AIDS virus is known as the Human Immunodeficiency Virus, or HIV. For AIDS infection to occur, a certain level of concentration of virus particles is necessary. This is discussed later in the book in relation to mosquito bites and deep kissing.

How it spreads
There has been much speculation and confusion over the way the AIDS virus spreads, which is one of the chief reasons why the disease is so feared. The speculation and confusion arose from lack of knowledge. At the beginning of the epidemic, medical scientists simply did not have enough information to be able to give reassuring answers.

Since then a great deal has been learned about the virus through research, and experience has accumulated through painstaking medical and epidemiological studies. It is now clear that HIV spreads primarily by sexual contact, both among male homosexuals and heterosexually. Unlike other sexually transmitted diseases, the virus is carried within semen, and it can also be carried by cervical and vaginal secretions, so that infection can be either from male to female or female to male. The greatest risk appears to be to the receptive partner in anal intercourse, because of the fragility of the lining of the rectum. The majority of AIDS cases in North America and Europe have so far occurred in homosexual men. But the virus also spreads through ordinary heterosexual intercourse. Most cases in Africa have occurred in this way, and the number occurring in North America and Europe is increasing.

Much has been made of the use of condoms to prevent AIDS infection. There is no doubt that condoms can offer some protection to passage of the AIDS virus. It has been shown in laboratory tests that the virus is unable to penetrate an intact latex condom, and there is evidence of reduction of infection rates among those practising so-called "safe sex." But to some extent "safe sex" is a misnomer, because condom failure *can* occur, just as it sometimes does when condoms are used for contraception (between five and 30 times out of 100 uses). Failures can also occur if condoms are improperly used, for example if semen should escape during withdrawal of the penis. The only truly safe sex is either abstinence from sexual intercourse (in which case it's not safe sex, it's no sex!) or sexual intercourse with a long-term partner known not to be HIV-infected. Other forms of sexual play, which do not involve penile penetration of the vagina or the anus, can also be safe from HIV infection, providing they do not involve the exchange of blood, semen or vaginal or cervical fluids. Deep kissing, involving exchange of saliva, has not been documented as causing HIV infection, but theoretically it could do so if there were breaks in the mucous membranes of the mouth.

Blood transfusions
Because the virus travels within the human body in blood, it can also be transmitted through the blood of an infected person. This occurs mainly in blood transfusions or through sharing of needles by intravenous drug users. Since November 1, 1985, the Canadian Red Cross has routinely been screening all blood donations for the AIDS virus antibody. The organization also asks donors not to give blood if they are in groups at

risk of being infected by the virus. These actions have greatly reduced the risk of being exposed to HIV infection through blood transfusion. The risk cannot be said to be zero, but it has been estimated to be less than one in a million — and may be considerably less than that depending on the efficiency of the screening tests. The extremely small risk that remains is due to the fact that screening tests obviously cannot show antibodies in the blood of persons so recently infected that they have not yet produced them. HIV antibodies appear as early as two to three weeks, or as late as five to six months after infection. Again, to put this level of risk in perspective, we must compare it with others we may undergo. In the case of a blood transfusion, it might be appropriate to compare it with the risk of dying from the effects of an anesthetic while in hospital, which is very small yet always present. In considering this risk, it is reassuring to know that, since 1985, *only two transfusion-associated cases of AIDS have been found in millions of U.S. recipients of blood screened for HIV antibody, and there have been none in Canada.*

Finally, the process of blood donation presents absolutely no risk of HIV infection to blood donors in Canada.

Canadians travelling to certain other countries may be at risk from contaminated blood supplies if they become injured and require a transfusion. Would-be travellers to areas where AIDS information is widespread are advised to inquire about precautions from their local public-health authorities.

Accidental exposure
Besides being found in semen and blood, the AIDS virus has been isolated from tears, vaginal and cervical secretions, cerebrospinal fluid and brain tissue. Theoretically, exposure to any of these could therefore present a risk of infection. But two factors have a bearing on whether infection actually takes place: one is the susceptibility of the individual, the other is the kind of exposure involved. What constitutes a susceptible individual is so far a mystery. There is evidence that susceptibility varies from person to person, but no one knows why this happens. Some think genetic factors may be responsible. The kind of exposure necessary for infection to occur is direct transfer of an infected body fluid through cuts, scratches, abrasions or broken mucous membranes. Intact skin provides complete protection. Cases have occurred of infection through skin puncture by needles or other sharp

objects, but none are known to have resulted from splashing or spilling of infected material onto intact membranes, such as those in the eyes or mouth. Nor is there any evidence for infection through swallowing or inhaling such fluids.

Despite the apparent dangers, the overall risk of infection in health-care workers is estimated at less than one percent in all those exposed. They are, in fact, more likely to get infections such as hepatitis B, which has a pattern of spread identical to HIV. This seems true even of dentists, who have frequent exposure to blood and saliva. In a study of 895 dental professionals, none of those who had reported that they were accidentally exposed to patients' blood had developed antibodies to HIV, whereas 22 percent of those who had not received the hepatitis-B vaccine had antibodies to the hepatitis-B virus. In Canada, a national surveillance program carried out since 1985 has shown none of the 120 health-care workers in the study who have been exposed to HIV-infected blood or body fluids have tested positive for the AIDS-virus antibody.

Can you get it from a toilet seat?
Casual contact with infected persons, insect bites or contact with inanimate objects such as toilet seats or doorknobs have never been found responsible for infection, despite several studies of the issue. Even prolonged, close (though non-sexual) household contact with persons with AIDS has shown no evidence of risk. In one study, those sharing toilets, baths, kitchens, dishes, eating utensils, combs and even toothbrushes, and who engaged in such close body contact as hugging and kissing, were not found to be at increased risk.

All this is not to say that infection *could not* occur under such circumstances, simply that if it has occurred, it has never been found to do so. On the other hand, it would be strange if studies such as those referred to did not uncover infections transmitted by such casual means if they had occurred. Hospital physicians will tell you that once certain other types of infection occur on a ward — say an infection of the mother after childbirth — it spreads like wildfire, yet this does not happen with AIDS.

The search for simple answers
Most people want a simple "yes" or "no" answer to a question like, "Can you get AIDS from a mosquito bite?" The problem is that the

situation usually cannot be described in black-and-white terms. This may go a long way towards explaining apparently different stories that appear in the media about how the disease is contracted.

Dr. Walter Dowdle, deputy director for AIDS at the U.S. Centers for Disease Control, illustrated such difficulties during a 1987 media seminar held by the Scientists' Institute for Public Information in Orlando, Florida.

"You all may recall this story," Dr. Dowdle told the media delegates. " 'Mosquitos Shown to Carry AIDS virus.' These stories reported that it was found that after a mosquito had a blood meal containing the AIDS virus, the virus was still present up to 48 hours later.

"But what does this really mean? It is true, of course, that mosquitos carry certain viral diseases, like yellow fever, in their salivary glands. What most of these reports didn't mention, however, was that the AIDS virus does not grow in the salivary gland; it is simply in the mosquito's gut. And generally after one blood meal, the mosquito will go off and rest until that meal is digested, thus digesting the AIDS virus as well.

"In order to construct a scenario for mosquito-transmitted AIDS infection, we must assume that, one, the mosquito first bites a person infected with the AIDS virus and then immediately bites someone else; two, while the second person was being bitten, the mosquito suddenly got sick and regurgitated on the second person's skin; three, the second person realized he was being bitten and slapped at the mosquito, thus rubbing the regurgitated virus into the wound left by the mosquito; and four, that virus would have to be about 1,000 to 10,000 times more concentrated than is ever found in anybody's blood.

"Now, this is obviously a very, very unlikely scenario. Your challenge is getting across the fact that while such a case — like so many incidents involving possible AIDS infection — may be possible, it is extraordinarily unlikely."

Because this question of whether or not it is possible to contact AIDS through casual contact seems to preoccupy most people, it is worth stressing that the *only infections so far have resulted from blood-to-blood or semen-blood transfer*. A related concern with large numbers of people is whether the virus can be passed through exchange of saliva, as in deep kissing, for example. Here it is worth quoting Dr. Alastair Clayton, director-general of Canada's Federal Centre for AIDS. "To get a high enough concentration of virus to produce infection," he says, "it has been calculated you'd need *four litres* of saliva. Even then, passing this amount from mouth to mouth wouldn't do it — the four litres would have to go straight into the bloodstream." (See also appendix, "Clinging to Misconceptions.)

From mother to child

The third main avenue of infection with AIDS is in many ways the most unfortunate: an infected pregnant woman can pass the virus to her infant. According to scientific evidence, this is done during pregnancy or during labour and delivery, not through household contact. The only known case in which the infection was contracted after birth is believed to have possibly occurred through the mother's milk, since the mother herself did not become HIV-positive until after her child was born. No other cases of infection through mother's milk have been recorded; in fact other children who have breast-fed from infected mothers have themselves remained uninfected, so this route may be rare. Yet the overall risk of infection of babies by AIDS-infected mothers is significant: from 17 percent to as high as 65 percent in different studies.

Other risk factors

Besides the possibility of variations in individual genetic susceptibility, certain other factors appear to play a role in determining who gets AIDS. Those who previously have had other sexually transmitted diseases seem to be at greater risk of AIDS, as do those who have had many sexual partners. (Regarding the latter, it is obvious that the greater the number of partners has been, the greater also has been the opportunity for AIDS infection.) Those who have previously suffered from other viral infections also appear to be at greater risk of AIDS.

How AIDS shows up and how it progresses

It usually takes from six to eight weeks after infection for HIV antibodies to show up in the blood. Yet, as with many other aspects of the disease, this latency period varies from person to person. It may take months or years for antibodies to show up, and there have actually been cases where they never have done so, although the virus itself has been cultured from the individual's blood.

Once the infection has been acquired, the course of the disease also varies from individual to individual. Some patients may have no symptoms at all to begin with, while others will suffer from an illness that resembles influenza or mononucleosis, with fever and generalized aches and pains. A large number suffer from lymphadenopathy, in which the lymph nodes in their neck, armpits and groin remain swollen for more than three months. (The nodes swell when they produce large numbers of white blood cells to fight infection.) Other patients suffer not just fever but also weight loss and diarrhea; dementia; or a wide variety of secondary diseases such as brain inflammation caused by a parasite called toxoplasmosis; herpes zoster (shingles); tuberculosis; or rare cancers such as Kaposi's sarcoma. These secondary diseases are able to take hold because the body's immune system has been weakened by the AIDS-virus infection.

How many of those infected by HIV will go on to develop full-blown AIDS, or over what period of time, is not known. Again there is great variability among individuals. Early in the epidemic, it was estimated that five to 10 percent of those infected would eventually develop AIDS, but as time went on these estimates rose to 20-30 percent and higher. Most authorities now believe that eventually all those infected will come down with the disease: at present AIDS has not been recognized long enought to tell. Recent results from a San Francisco study, in which the date of infection was fairly well established, estimated the probability of developing AIDS as five percent after three years, 10 percent after four years, 15 percent after five years, 24 percent after six years, 31 percent after seven years, and 36 percent after seven-and-a-half years. A Canadian study has shown similar estimates.

Testing for HIV infection
The surest way to determine whether an individual is carrying the AIDS virus would be to recover the virus itself from blood, body fluids or tissue. While this is technically possible, it is too expensive, time-consuming and difficult to do routinely. In fact, the techniques are available only in a few centres in Canada.

Instead, the procedures currently used routinely test for *antibody* to the AIDS virus. Two types are used, one for screening and the other for confirming screening test results. What they show, it must be remembered, is simply that the body has responded to the presence of the AIDS virus by producing antibody. They do not show how infective the individual is, or whether he or she will utimately go on to develop the AIDS disease. As noted above, the risk of developing the disease increases with time among those infected, but there have been rare reports of a very small number of individuals who originally showed a positive result to testing later showing a negative response. The reason for this is not known, but it suggests either that the original test result was faulty or that somehow the body was able to fight off the disease. If the latter were true it would have important implications, but the number of cases involved is too small to allow conclusions to be drawn. So for the time being these cases remain mysteries.

It is important to note that the presence of AIDS virus antibodies in a person's bloodstream does not necessarily mean that person is a carrier of live AIDS virus. There is a *theoretical* possibility that an individual might show antibody to HIV in a blood test without actually being infected by the virus: the antibodies could be produced in response to dead or inactive virus particles. This is what happens with Salk polio vaccine: the virus in the vaccine, which was killed when the vaccine was made, stimulated the body to produce antibodies in the absence of any infection. Using the methods routinely employed for HIV testing, it would be impossible to determine whether the antibodies produced resulted from live or dead viruses.

Important implications follow from this for the development of an AIDS vaccine. For if an AIDS vaccine makes a person test positive for AIDS antibodies, how could those involved in vaccine trials be distinguished from individuals who are truly HIV-infected? Identification cards have been proposed for those involved in the trials to say that their positive HIV status does not indicate that they are necessarily AIDS-virus carriers. But who believes that such a device would protect such persons against discrimination?

A full discussion of the use of blood tests in AIDS, and their implications, will be found in Chapter Three.

Treatment and prevention

Unfortunately, there is no cure for AIDS, and no really effective treatment. Doctors can treat the secondary infections with varying degrees of success, but not the underlying AIDS infection. These treatments can help make the patient more comfortable, and perhaps lengthen life, but they cannot get rid of the AIDS virus or prevent the ultimate fate of the patient. A number of drugs and treatments to fight the AIDS virus and bolster the patient's immune system are being used, but progress is slow. Large-scale efforts are also going on to develop a vaccine, but success seems years away — if in fact it can ever be achieved. One of the chief difficulties standing in the way of a vaccine is the ability of the HIV to mutate quickly, changing the proteins on its coat and thus making it difficult for body cells to recognize. Through this evasive tactic, the virus can always stay ahead of the immune system's antibodies, which have to identify the proteins of the virus to neutralize it. And since a vaccine works by stimulating production of appropriate antibodies in the body, it is helpless if the appropriate antibodies cannot be recognized.

AIDS in Canada: past, present and future
The first two cases of people with AIDS disease were officially reported in Canada during the first six months of 1982. Nine more were reported during the next six months. Then followed a period of near-exponential increase, with the number of cases doubling every eight to 10 months during 1983 and 1984. Since then the doubling time has decreased and the epidemic curve is no longer exponential, but the number of new cases has continued to rise dramatically, reaching 1,765 by May 24, 1988. Of these, 1,732 were adults and 33 were children. Ninety-four percent of all cases were males.

The first AIDS case was diagnosed in Montreal and initially the epidemic was concentrated there. Until 1984, Quebec reported the majority of cases. Since then, the rates for Ontario and British Columbia have increased more sharply, thus resulting in a proportionate decrease in the contribution from Quebec. By May, 1988, Ontario had the majority of diagnosed cases (689), followed by Quebec (529) and British Columbia (352).

Most cases early in the epidemic were from Montreal, Toronto and Vancouver (78 percent between 1979-82). But by 1984, the percentage of total cases in these three cities had dropped below 70 percent, and by 1987 to 62 percent. In 1987, 25 percent of the total came from cities with populations of 100,000 and over, and 13 percent were from elsewhere. Thus AIDS is increasingly becoming a problem in all Canada.

The majority of people with AIDS in Canada are in their most productive years: 90 percent are between age 20 and 49, with 47 percent between 30 and 39. Approximately 52 percent die in the year following diagnosis, 74 percent within two years. The social significance of the incidence figures therefore exceeds the numbers themselves.

In Canada as elsewhere, those with AIDS can be classified into groups, although the incidence of the disease among these groups differs from that in other countries. In Canada, 82 percent of persons with AIDS are homosexual/bisexual men; five percent are heterosexuals from regions where the disease is endemic, such as Haiti and Central Africa; 4.6 percent are recipients of blood transfusions; 2.4 percent are heterosexuals who have had sexual contact with a partner in a high-risk group, such as a bisexual or a person from an endemic region; 1.7 percent are hemophiliacs; and only 0.6 percent are intravenous drug abusers. Three percent could not be identified with any of these groups, but this may have been for lack of information.

HIV infection estimates
At present it is difficult if not impossible to estimate the total number of HIV-infected persons in Canada as opposed to those with diagnosed AIDS. Only parts of the picture are apparent.

AIDS in Quebec was initially concentrated in the Haitian community, but its spread within this community later slowed down. The estimated number of Haitians in Quebec who were HIV-infected in early 1988 was 1,600. Dramatic increases occurred more recently among Canadian homosexual/bisexuals: in early 1988 it was estimated that 20-40 percent of sexually active homosexual men were HIV-infected. Other estimates are that:

- 915 recipients of blood-clotting factors (hemophiliacs) have HIV.
- Some 600 women have become infected through heterosexual contact with either a clotting-factor recipient, a person from an area where AIDS is endemic or an IV drug user.
- Some 200 individuals became infected through contaminated blood before the Red Cross instituted screening methods.

The majority of HIV-infected Canadians may be unaware of their condition because they either have no symptoms at all or only swollen glands, which can, of course, occur for other reasons and may not take them to their doctor for diagnosis. Surveillance of the disease in Canada has relied on diagnostic criteria that apply to the condition known as full-blown AIDS, which gives an incomplete picture.

The AIDS total in Canada: less than expected?
As of September, 1987, the best available estimate of the total number of people in Canada infected with the AIDS virus, whether or not they show symptoms, is about 30,000, although the number could be as low as 10,000 or as high as 50,000. This is lower than previous estimates that have appeared widely in various documents, including the media, which ranged from 75,000 to 100,000.

Uncertainty has surrounded such estimates — and continues to do so — because the data necessary for precise incidence figures are simply not available. No systematic blood testing of the general population has been carried out, and the data from the provinces cannot be relied upon because of what is known as the "volunteer effect": since the tests are done on those who have volunteered to have them, they do not give a true picture of the situation as a whole. The reason the latest estimate (30,000) is lower than previous ones is because of the way in which such estimates are arrived at. Epidemiologists use what they term the *infected-to-AIDS* ratio for this purpose. This represents the number of individuals within the population who have been infected by HIV at a certain point in time, divided by the number who have actually developed AIDS at the same point. The inclusion of a time reference is important because the ratio will change with time, the reason being the lag between infection and the appearance of the illness. Early in the epidemic, when the number of full-blown AIDS cases was small, the ratio was extremely large. But as time goes on the ratio falls dramatically. For example, in San Francisco among 6,700 homosexual men recruited in 1978 for a hepatitis-B study, 275 were later found to have HIV-positive blood although none had AIDS, making the infected-to-AIDS ratio infinite. Two years later the infected-to-AIDS ratio had risen to an estimated 825:1, while by 1984 it had fallen to 28:1.

This ratio provides an easy way to estimate the number of infected individuals in a population: you simply multiply the ratio by the number of individuals who have developed AIDS. For example, in 1984, the number of infected individuals in the United States was estimated at between 500,000 and one million by multiplying the estimated infected-to-AIDS ratio of between 50:1 and 100:1 by the number of observed AIDS cases, 10,000.

Unfortunately, few recent calculations take into account the fact that these ratios are likely to have fallen since 1984; in 1987, people were still making calculations on the basis of an infected-to-AIDS ratio of as high as 100:1. This has likely caused an overestimation of the true number of AIDS cases. In 1987, most Canadian media still referred to a figure of 50,000-100,000 infected Canadians that probably originated from the use of an infected-to-AIDS ratio of between 50:1 and 100:1 during a period when roughly 1,000 AIDS cases had been reported.

Epidemiologists use mathematical models to predict the future course of the epidemic. Different models produce different predictions. Using two different models, Royal Society of Canada epidemiologists have forecast that the cumulative number of AIDS cases in Canada will total between 6,000 and 11,000 by 1992. The implications of these figures will be discussed in the next chapter.

CHAPTER TWO

AIDS In Perspective

When confronted with the problems posed by AIDS, most people tend to feel overwhelmed — and with good reason. Here is an infectious and incurable disease that, once established, leads in the vast majority of cases to unusual, extremely painful conditions against which both the human body's natural defences and all the sophisticated weapons of modern medicine are powerless. Then, in a matter usually of a year or two, AIDS invariably and inexorably results in death.

That is the fate of those diagnosed with full-blown Acquired Immunodeficiency Syndrome. But even those shown by blood tests to be carriers of the Human Immunodeficiency Virus, or HIV, find themselves in a highly uncertain situation. They may appear to be and feel perfectly well, and without symptoms of any kind. They may remain well for years. Whether any AIDS-virus carriers will escape the disease is not yet known. As noted in the last chapter, most authorities now expect *all* those infected with HIV will succumb to it eventually. The outcome is uncertain because AIDS has not been around long enough — or at least has not been recognized long enough — for medical scientists to understand the course of the disease.

As a result of all this, fear of AIDS has become widespread among Canadians. To some extent, certainly, the fear is well-founded. But in some ways it is an unreasoning fear that has reached the point where it could easily turn to panic. Some indication that this has already happened appears in the calls that have been made for unnecessary and useless quarantine and discrimination against AIDS carriers.

A sense of proportion
What is needed to prevent this panic reaction from spreading is a sense of proportion. First of all, we need to recognize that safety from risks is relative, an apparently obvious fact that nevertheless seems often to be overlooked in these days of consumerism and political activism. None of us can avoid all risk: as someone once put it, "Living is

dangerous to your health.'' Or, as the organizing committee of a Royal Society of Canada symposium on the assessment and perception of risk to human health in Canada in 1982 pointed out, ''Absolute safety is an illusion.'' It noted that comparisons can help people understand the difficult mathematics of risk. Quoting E. Pochin, from the *Journal of the Royal College of Physicians* (Vol. 12, No. 3, April, 1978), the committee listed the following activities as posing a one-in-a-million chance of death:

- travelling 400 miles by air
- travelling 60 miles by car
- smoking three-quarters of a cigarette
- rock climbing for 1½ minutes
- engaging in typical factory work for 1½ weeks
- being a man aged 60 for 20 minutes

The committee also noted that comparison of mortality statistics with perceptions of risk has shown that ''there is a tendency by the public to overestimate some of the less-frequent causes. It is well known in scientific circles that some risks are associated with needlessly exaggerated fears . . . .''

This was illustrated in a table published in *Science*, the journal of the American Association for the Advancement of Science, on April 17, 1987, as part of a Risk Assessment issue. The table showed that the League of Women Voters and college students rated nuclear power as the most risky of a number of factors, while nuclear experts, who presumably knew more about the subject, rated it only 20th in order of riskiness. On the other hand, the League of Women Voters rated contraceptives 20th on their list, while college students listed them 9th and experts 11th.

Perception of risk

The British Medical Association guide *Living With Risk* notes that the more available is information on a given event, the more likely people will judge it to occur:

Things which really do happen often are, of course, easy to bring to mind, but many other factors also influence recall. These include the regular reporting of events which are not truly very frequent, and exposure to dramatic information which is rich in death and disaster. A helicopter crashed into the North Sea in 1986 with the sad death of nearly all the oil rig workers it was carrying. Cries followed for new and more stringent safety measures for helicopters, because of the immediate perception that they 'must be' dangerous aircraft. But in 1985 there was not a single fatal helicopter crash in the U.K., and only six large helicopters were reported to have crashed fatally in the entire world, which would seem in fact to indicate an extraordinarily low degree of risk in helicopter operation. The book *Jaws* was about leaders of a community who wanted to suppress news that a shark was in the vicinity so as to *decrease* the perceived risk, in order that tourists might not be discouraged. In the real world, publication of the book stimulated to an unprecedented extent the fear of sharks which already existed throughout the world.

A study by psychologists in Oregon showed that people tended to overestimate the incidence of rare cause of death — the very ones most reported in newspapers — and underestimate the frequency of common ones. The same researchers noted that people may well not be reassured by being told that rare events are indeed rare. For example, if an engineer were to stress the safety of a power plant by describing its safety features in detail, people might feel that if so many features were needed to make it safe, it simply proved that the plant was dangerous.

Another factor that affects people's perceptions of risk is the so-called "dread factor," which characterizes events that are out of personal control, have potentially catastrophic consequences on a global scale with fatal outcomes, are evenly distributed, pose a high risk to future generations, are increasing and not easily reduced, are involuntary and have potential to affect the individual. The higher an activity rates on the dread factor, the greater is its perceived risk, and the more people want to see it reduced — and the more they want to see strict regulation employed to achieve this. Obviously, the dread factor would rate very high in AIDS in most people's opinions.

Some comparisons
Perception of risk is clearly a very complex matter, depending to a large extent on personal biases and the context of a particular risk in society. Statistics are not the only factor involved in risk perception (we will deal with others in Chapter Four), yet in assessing risk we must use some

standard of comparison. One way of putting the AIDS threat in perspective, then, is to examine its position as a risk nationally and internationally, compared with other diseases. For example, the 1,464 *total cases* of AIDS that were reported in Canada in the *five years* between 1982 and 1987 compare with 47,407 *deaths* from heart disease in only *one year* (1985, the latest for which Statistics Canada figures are available). So far in Canada, only 984 people have died from AIDS (May, 1988). And in the entire world, only 80,912 cases of AIDS had been reported by March, 1988. While it is true that the number of AIDS cases worldwide is believed to be much higher than reported (between five and ten million people are estimated to be infected with the AIDS virus, and between half a million and three million are expected to die from it by 1991), when compared with *other* causes of death the AIDS numbers look small. For example, malaria kills some 400 million people each year worldwide, hepatitis-B virus and schistosomiasis (snail fever) kill 200 million, and both tuberculosis (with three million deaths) and leprosy (with two million) still are greater threats to mankind than is AIDS.

Because AIDS is preventable, its incidence should be compared with other preventable diseases, and when this is done we see that other preventable diseases occur on a much larger scale. For example, in Canada heart disease is the leading cause of death. Cancer runs a close second: in 1985, 46,333 Canadians died from cancer, which was the leading cause of death in Quebec, Alberta and British Columbia. Today it is recognized that deaths from both heart disease and cancer can be reduced by changes in lifestyle and other factors. Since 1955, when heart foundations in Canada came into existence, Statistics Canada figures show that the number of deaths from all cardiovascular diseases in this country has been reduced by 36 percent. Similarly, there has been a 28 percent reduction in the death rate from heart attacks, 50 percent in the case of strokes, 87 percent in rheumatic heart disease and 88 percent in high blood pressure.

It has been estimated that some 70 percent of cancers are caused by environmental factors, and therefore, theoretically at least, are avoidable. Death from lung cancer among males numbered 8,278 in 1985 and 3,164 among females. The chief cause of lung cancer is cigarette smoking — an entirely voluntary activity. Cirrhosis of the liver linked to alcohol consumption killed 591 men and 191 women. Two hundred and eighty men and 207 women died of malignant melanoma, which is partly linked to exposure to the sun — also largely voluntary. And 2,980 men and 1,254 women died in motor-vehicle accidents.

Risk probabilities

Another way of looking at health risks is to ask what is the probability of contracting a disease. The Canadian Cancer Society, in *Canadian Cancer Statistics 1987*, estimated, for the first time, the probability of an individual Canadian developing a particular form of cancer, assuming current incidence and death rates. The conclusion was that just over one in three Canadians will develop *some form* of cancer during their lifetime, while the probability of developing certain types of cancer ranges between five percent and 10 percent. By comparison, the probability that a Canadian will die from an accident is six percent in males and four percent in females, and from suicide is 1.4 percent in males and 0.6 percent in females. Similar probabilities for AIDS would be extremely difficult to work out because the number of victims is currently so small. But the probability of a Canadian dying from AIDS is obviously far less than the already extremely small likelihood of dying by suicide, because while 886 Canadians have died from AIDS in the last five years, 3,249 took their own lives in 1985 alone.

AIDS as an avoidable disease

AIDS seems particularly frightening because once infected with the AIDS virus, victims apparently remain infected for life, a large percentage will go on to develop the full-blown disease, and there is no cure or even satisfactory treatment. But unlike most risks, AIDS for the majority of people is *almost completely avoidable*. It is caused by a virus spread almost exclusively in three ways: sexual contact with an infected person, sharing of needles by intravenous drug users and transfusions of infected blood. Since blood transfusions now are screened for the virus and are therefore almost free of risk, and excepting transmission of the virus from mother to baby before or during birth, there are really only two ways: sexual contact and needle sharing. Both of these are avoidable, except in cases of sexual assault or deception by an infected sexual partner. (A few accidents have occurred in laboratories, but again, these are avoidable.)

There is absolutely no evidence that the AIDS virus can be spread by casual contact with an infected person (for example by living in the same house and sharing cooking utensils and bathroom facilities). And there is much inferential evidence that this *does not* happen; for example, no incident has been recorded in which AIDS has been passed from food handlers in San Francisco, despite the fact that that city contains the greatest concentration of AIDS cases in North America, and despite the fact that a proportion of its food handlers are known to be members of high-risk groups.

Thus, barring extremely unlikely accidents, anyone who wants to avoid contracting AIDS can do so. All they need do is either avoid sexual contact with another person altogether (an unlikely solution for many) or maintain a long-standing monogamous sexual relationship, and avoid the use of non-sterilized needles for intravenous injection. Theoretically, therefore, we have within our grasp the means to stem the currently rapid spread of AIDS.

Demanding that others protect us
Whether the risk of contracting AIDS is a voluntary one or one to which we are subjected involuntarily is an important point, which has a bearing on the increasing demands we are hearing to make AIDS testing of certain groups mandatory. As was discussed in Chapter One, AIDS tests are not entirely reliable, a fact that argues against their widespread mandatory use. But apart from that, such demands probably stem to a great extent from a phenomenon described at the aforementioned Royal Society of Canada risk symposium by Stuart L. Smith, then chairman of the Science Council of Canada.

Smith, who is a psychiatrist, noted that the psychology of risk is such that, ''when it lies within the power of *others* to protect us, then we sometimes overrate the risk probability and we demand protection by those in a position to offer it.

Take, for example, crime in the streets,'' said Smith. ''If you are an average person, whether he or she is seriously at risk of being mugged or murdered on a Toronto street, they will say, 'Yes, look at all the murders, look at the rapes, look how terrible things are.' The fact is that the real likelihood of this happening to an individual is extremely low . . . . The real chances of being murdered in the street are just negligible compared to the odds of being killed by an automobile or dying of natural causes at any given moment. And yet people think they are at serious risk, they demand greater police protection every time they hear of someone who was unfortunate enough to have suffered that particular fate . . . . Yet when it lies mainly within *our own power to protect ourselves*, we frequently *fail to do so.* When we think it's up to someone else to protect us, we demand full protection, but when we have it within our own power, we often do not use it. This is a fundamental aspect of the public's perception with respect to risks. We seem to find a risk more acceptable than a change in our personal lifestyle or a change in our self-perception. I give as examples, automobile driving habits, smoking and the non-use of respiratory protectors at work.

Smith's comments were made before the current concern about AIDS, so he could not have had this risk in mind. Yet they are highly relevant to the current situation. What may well be behind many demands for AIDS testing is just what he describes — a demand for others to protect us when we perceive (realistically or not) that it is within their power to do so, when in fact we are capable of protecting ourselves.

Who is ultimately responsible?
Looked at in light of the above, our perception of the AIDS threat may well change. We see that there are certain things that others can do to protect us and thus protect society as a whole, but there are some things only we can do for ourselves. The primary responsibility in limiting the spread of AIDS belongs to each member of society. AIDS testing, segregation of those infected with virus, adoption and enforcement of restrictions in the name of public health — all these may or may not help combat the epidemic (a question that will be discussed in later chapters). What will be the determining factor will be each individual's actions to protect him or her self from infection. Segregation of AIDS-infected people will not allow those not infected to continue a risk-free, liberated sex life, and to believe this is to deceive ourselves. Nor will such actions protect one's children.

AIDS and sexual values
In a very real way, then, the AIDS epidemic has revived what used to be considered moral, ethical or religious questions related to sexual conduct. Today the same considerations may apply, but in a biological context. If we wish, the traditional values of chastity or exclusivity of

sexual partners can now be argued from the point of view of biological benefit or disbenefit to the individual and to society as a whole, rather than on the basis of morality, ethics or religion. How each person answers these questions remains an individual decision, but answer them we must. AIDS has marked *finis* to the holiday many of us took from making sexual value judgments in the Age of Aquarius.

In a society whose sexual mores are predominantly liberal, this is not going to be easy. Older members of society have only just overcome the suffocating suppression and hypocritical aspects of Victorianism. Will young people particularly, who have known only sexual freedom, take readily to the new situation? Hedonism is a much more predominant part of today's society than is self-discipline. What kinds of restrictions, self-imposed or otherwise, are young people of both sexes willing to accept? The only thing that may make their decision easier is that young people are the group at greatest risk.

Yet the world of the young offers much hope. Physical exercise is in vogue among them, and light wines and beers much more popular than whisky. Their political action groups are highly visible, pitted with almost evangelical fervour against every modern evil from environmental pollution to militarism. Although the fever days of the '60s campus rebels are long gone, no university president is heard today bemoaning the excessive conformity of his students and pleading with them, as Sidney Smith did at the University of Toronto in the '50s: "Characters, your country needs you."

Looking backwards

In grappling with modern problems, the lessons of history are sometimes helpful. AIDS is not the first pandemic. So what can we learn from the past?

Unfortunately not much, because in a number of ways AIDS is unique. When the most terrible of all epidemic diseases of antiquity, the Black Death, struck Europe in the 14th century, those who became victims could almost immediately be seen as such, because the disease quickly manifested itself. The plague was caused by a bacillus conveyed to man by a flea that infested rats, and the incubation period was only a few days. After that the disease set in suddenly with fever, headache, lassitude and aching of the limbs. Victims suffered temperatures of 103 degrees or more, their skin was hot and dry, their tongue furred and they became insatiably thirsty. The lymph glands of plague sufferers also swelled visibly (the "bubos" of bubonic plague). The sunken eyes, stupor and sometimes wild delirium that followed left no doubt in the minds of onlookers as to what had happened.

Similarly short incubation periods occur in other epidemics, for example influenza, and the symptoms are also easily identified. With AIDS, symptoms may not appear for weeks, months or years; doctors still do not know how long the dormancy can last.

Detention
In the past, quarantine was often used to detain those who returned from areas where disease was widespread until it could be determined whether or not they had contracted it. This usually could be done within 40 days (from which comes the term "quarantine") because of the short incubation period. With AIDS, the incubation period is unknown, and quarantine is unnecessary because those infected with HIV can be identified with blood tests. There is no point in detaining them because the disease is not contagious in the sense the ancient diseases were, and because in any case HIV infection is already spread throughout the world and all of us live in infected regions.

Leprosy and tuberculosis have never assumed epidemic proportions in Canada, but they are diseases whose social aspects can be compared to AIDS. The very name "leper" implies the outcast from society, and while the disease has largely been eliminated from Western countries, it still flourishes in some developing ones. The leper still is kept apart from society, despite the fact that his condition is one of the least contagious of communicable diseases. Tubercular patients as recently as the 1930s were whisked away to sanatoriums outside urban areas and isolated from the rest of society, in what may seem in hindsight to have been as much an attempt to hide their problem as to solve it. Unlike both leprosy and AIDS, TB is in fact highly contagious in the sense that it can spread by droplets of saliva. A certain percentage of the population is always infected but may remain well and symptom-free all their lives, probably succumbing to the disease only if they become highly stressed, badly nourished and run-down.

Can science conquer AIDS?
The omnipresence of the infectious organisms in our environment, which in these days of antibiotics is often forgotten, may help to put AIDS fears into perspective. Despite our modern miracle drugs, disease

is not something that is "conquered" by man. It is always with us. The infective organisms are not wiped off the face of the earth; they remain always present in the environment to a greater or lesser degree. For some we have effective drugs that will kill an invasion in most patients. Others become resistant, as has happened with gonorrhea, so that new antibiotics have to be developed in a constant battle against the causative organisms. The war against disease is a continuing one. New drugs, like new weapons in conventional combat, can win individual battles and even turn the tide of the fight from time to time, but the war goes on. Despite even these powerful weapons, battles are sometimes lost in individuals whose bodies — or whose wills — have become weakened sufficently for a disease to take hold and overcome both natural and artificial defences.

Similarities with syphilis

Is it possible that mankind and the AIDS virus could somehow reach a kind of equilibrium, in which the disease would remain among us without actually decimating us? It is too early to tell. We have not yet contained it, as we did with smallpox. And the AIDS virus has the incomparable advantage of attacking and taking over for its own reproduction the body's own defence system — the immune system. Yet it is possible we can contain AIDS without actually eliminating it completely. This containment is what has happened with the disease that affords the closest parallel with AIDS: syphilis. Despite continual surveillance and effective drugs, syphilis remains with us. The massive educational programs that were mounted to contain the spread of venereal diseases in Canada had mixed results, according to Jay Cassel's historical narrative, *The Secret Plague, Venereal Disease in Canada 1838-1939* (University of Toronto Press). In that period, he writes,

> many improvements were made in the treatment and control of VD. Understanding of the diseases was greatly increased. Diagnosis and treatment were much improved. After years of inaction, Canadians set up a system that provided treatment for anyone in need and made information available to everyone. It took a long time to come that far, and yet there was still a problem. Like many elements in the human condition, sexual health has not been vastly improved by a bold, simple step.

With the introduction of penicillin in 1943, hopes were high that syphilis and gonorrhea would finally be eliminated. Indeed the incidence fell sharply at first.

Then in the late 1950s a disturbing thing happened: the incidence of VD began to rise again. The increase in syphilis was moderate, and in the 1970s it levelled off, albeit unevenly. Gonorrhea, always more of a problem, rose at an alarming rate, establishing itself as the most common bacterial infection in humans. Moreover, many other sexually transmitted diseases were identified, and their incidence was also increasing. In the midst of this unpleasant trend, doctors began to encounter strains of the microorganisms causing syphilis and gonorrhea that were resistant to the new drugs. Evidently the situation in the early antibiotic era was not as good as it might at first appear.

Cassel concludes that sexually transmitted diseases remain a problem, in large part because of the importance of sex in people's lives:

> In an age when many things impinge on the individual and on freedom of action, the need for sex at a most basic personal level is obviously strong. It will not be easy to persuade people to limit their sexual activity because it *may* lead to infection . . . . Given these intensely personal considerations, many individuals simply will not do as they are advised or obliged to do, no matter how much medical sense it may make.

AIDS's exceptional ability
Of the striking differences that exist between the great epidemics of the past and the AIDS outbreak, perhaps the most important is a physical characteristic of the causative organism: the virus's ability literally to take over the defence mechanisms of the body. As noted in Chapter One, the story of the Trojan horse comes to mind, but in AIDS not only does the virus, like the invading soldiers inside the horse, gain surreptitious access to the stronghold of the body's defence system, it manages to convert the defending army into copies of itself. Because the invader assumes the identity of the invaded, medical science is powerless to strike at the one without harming the other. And as though this insulting tactic were not enough, the virus can, even before gaining access to the cells of its victims, change its identity with lightning speed — 1,000 times more quickly than that of the influenza virus,

with whose myriad disguises researchers have been unable to keep pace in making vaccines.

Another difference between the AIDS epidemic and those of the past is that none of its predecessors has occurred in a world so replete with information systems. These ensure that every new discovery about the disease is instantly disseminated worldwide to scientist and layman alike. While this has its positive features, it also has unfortunate aspects, because along with all the valid new information come rumours, scares and false alarms. To a public already alarmed, the result can be highly confusing, even terrifying. How can we separate facts and informed opinion from misinformation and even hogwash?

The real lessons of the past

What we can learn from historical precedents of AIDS is the tremendous potential for irrational cruelty that human contagion brings with it. In the days of the plague, the disease was commonly thought to be caused by the wrath of God (just as some today see divine retribution in the AIDS epidemic). Guided by this belief, terrified crowds then massacred those who represented sin in their deviation from accepted physical or social norms: Jews, strangers, village idiots and "witches." Some, though not massacred, were dragged into fields and left there to die.

Victims of plague, leprosy and tuberculosis have all suffered from social ostracism in various ways and to various degrees. Yet their isolation from the rest of humanity did little or nothing, in itself, to stem the spread of these diseases. In the case of the plague, isolation served some purpose in helping to contain its spread when the epidemic was at its height, because the disease was so highly contagious, but it was the elimination of rats and their parasites, fleas, from human dwellings that really prevented the widespread recurrence of the disease. Abject living conditions similarly are at the heart of the problem of leprosy; isolating patients keeps their misery from the eyes of others, but does little to prevent those others from becoming lepers themselves. And the decline in the TB death rate came *before* the advent of TB sanatoriums, again as a result of improvements in the poor living conditions involved in causing the disease.

The medieval persecution of victims of past epidemics today seems to us appalling. We think of the perpetrators of these actions as ignorant, superstitious, benighted people. But how much difference is there really from some current attitudes? A prominent American columnist proposed tattooing of AIDS carriers. Others have pressed for the exclusion from school of children with AIDS. Books have been written containing arguments that only thinly disguise an underlying moral abhorrence of homosexuality and the use of illicit drugs. Whatever we might think of such practices, are we in danger of persecuting groups who indulge in them in the guise of protecting society? We must be very sure that such proposals as widespread AIDS testing and segregation of AIDS sufferers will really have a positive effect on the spread of the disease before we advocate them. We must also consider what effects such actions might have on those who became infected through such non-sexual means as blood transfusions or during birth. If we are truly concerned with stopping the spread of the disease and caring for those who already have it, concepts of guilt and innocence will have no part to play in the measures we take. Such considerations are discussed in later chapters.

Because of the enormous uncertainty surrounding so many aspects of the AIDS epidemic, perhaps the most useful thing Canadians can do is concentrate their energies not on trying to control potential carriers of the disease, or blaming them, but rather on caring for the sick. In this way we would make sure we do not simply abandon them. Lawyers and sociologists have already sensed the impending potential for discrimination and cruelty in this epidemic, as we shall see later on. If we as citizens recognize such problems before they arise, perhaps we can show the basic humanitarianism of our society by trying to work out how best we can repond to sick individuals in terms of care,cost and justice. For a civilized society, helping the doomed to die with dignity is as important as trying to ensure the safety of those who have, so far, escaped their fate.

CHAPTER THREE

The Testing Dilemma

The development of tests purporting to show that a person has been infected by the AIDS virus might seem at first glance to be a tremendous boon to doctors, patients and society at large. Doctors and patients presumably would welcome such tests to help treat or cure the disease, and society would benefit from having AIDS-infected people educated about how to stem its spread. In fact, society *has* benefited from testing, for example in ensuring a safe blood supply for transfusions. But the availability of AIDS tests has, in addition, forced upon all of us one of the central dilemmas surrounding the disease, a dilemma that has caused much mental agony to doctors and policymakers over decisions about whether and when to test, and to individuals over whether or not to be tested. To understand this problem, we have to consider the nature of AIDS, the lack of useful treatments for it, the limitations of the tests, and the consequences of identifying those who have been infected.

First of all, infection by the AIDS virus does not show up for a matter of weeks or months, so that any test to reveal infection must be administered that long after exposure. A more recent infection by the virus will not show up, and infection may also occur after testing has been done. Secondly, there is no effective treatment available and no cure for AIDS, so that *knowing* whether or not one has been infected does not offer any advantage to the person taking the test — except perhaps relief of anxiety (about which more later). On the other hand, if other people learn an individual has been infected, the consequences to that person can be catastrophic: they may include the loss of a spouse or the disruption of a close sexual relationship, the loss of a job, the inability to obtain a mortgage or an insurance policy, or disruption of close friendships and even family relationships. So serious have the potential consequences seemed to some who have found themselves HIV-positive that they have thought of suicide — and others have actually sought that way out. Finally, there are little-publicized but inherent uncertainties involved in the tests themselves.

The real purpose of tests

Medicine is an art as well as a science. When a patient goes to the doctor with reasons to believe he or she might have a disease, the doctor begins the diagnosis by "taking a medical history." This involves listening to the patient and asking questions. Depending upon how well the doctor knows the patient, such questions may just not be about present symptoms, but about past illnesses, family background, health habits and other pertinent data. Only after that may the doctor call for tests. The tests are ordered as an *aid* to diagnosis — not to make the diagnosis itself. It's not like putting a car up on a ramp, attaching electrodes that feed into a computer and presto! a diagnosis. People are more complicated than cars, and so are diseases and their manifestations. The doctor decides what he or she thinks is wrong through a complex process of investigation that may or not include laboratory tests, and that does not rely solely on the tests to do the job.

All blood tests are subject to error, and the AIDS blood tests are no exception. It is perhaps less than generally understood that science deals mostly in probabilities rather than absolutes. Blood tests indicate the *probability* that a person has a certain condition. How accurate they are depends on many things, including the way the test are designed, the skill and experience of those carrying them out and the way the results are interpreted. How reliably a given test can indicate the presence of a disease is partly determined by the proportion of individuals in a population who *have* that disease. Generally speaking, the smaller the number of AIDS cases in a given population, the less reliable is the test in identifying infected individuals within it. This means that most antibody tests in a population in which an infection is uncommon would yield false positives. There are obvious implications for a disease with such a low incidence as AIDS in Canada.

ELISA and the Western Blot

The test used for AIDS screening is called ELISA (enzyme-linked immunosorbent assay). It is inexpensive, rapid and easy to use. It is highly sensitive, meaning that it will seldom fail to identify persons who actually have antibody, but this asset is counterbalanced by a weakness:

it is not very specific, meaning that it is likely to show false positive results. Furthermore, the rate of false positives varies from one commercial kit to another, and even among different batches of the same company's kit.

In populations with a low prevalence of AIDS, the ELISA tests produce *many* false positives. For example, the prevalence of infection among Canadian Red Cross blood donors has been found to be less than 0.02 percent — and as a result *more than 90 percent* of ELISA tests in this group prove to be false positives. This is not so bad as it sounds, because the reason the Red Cross is testing is to make sure no AIDS virus gets into its transfusion blood supply, where it can infect recipients, so it is wise to have a test that errs on the side of caution. In fact, the ELISA test was developed specifically for transfusion screening. But because it yields so many false positives, *any* positive result from an ELISA test calls for a repeat of the test — sometimes not just once but twice to make sure. And even after that a different kind of test called the Western Blot analysis is used for confirmation. A confirmation from the Western Blot test is taken as proof that the person who tested positive with ELISA is actually infected with the AIDS virus.

Yet the Western Blot test, too, has its uncertainties. It is not a standardized commercial product like the ELISA test, and its performance may vary substantially from one laboratory to another. An inexperienced laboratory's ability to do the test may be much less than an experienced one's, perhaps even unacceptably low. Fortunately for Canadians, this is less likely to happen than in the United States, where commercial laboratories may be involved, because Western Blot tests are carried out only in provincial laboratories under standardized conditions. Furthermore, if the results of a Western Blot test are uncertain, it will be carried out a second time using more accurate techniques at the Federal Centre for AIDS in Ottawa. But this does not provide certainty; even using the series of ELISA and Western Blot tests, as is done in Canada, can produce false positives. Among female blood donors in this country, where the prevalence of infection is extremely low (less than 0.01 percent), this sequence of tests may still be correct only part of the time. This is because the likelihood of obtaining false positives is much higher among low-risk populations than among high-risk ones.

The importance of interpretation

We can see how the interpretation of ELISA results can vary by looking at the operation of the test itself. The test uses proteins from AIDS virus first grown in tissue culture and then coated in wells on large plates, or on beads. The blood sample is added to the well or exposed to the beads. If the sample has antibodies in it, they bind to the virus and are detected through a colour reaction quantified by a spectrophotometer or by eye. The higher the level of antibody in the sample, the stronger the colour reaction. But since the results are measured on a continuous numerical scale, the test evaluator has to decide which values are to be deemed "positive" and which "negative." The threshold or cutoff point will determine how many false positives and false negatives there will be.

Since ELISA tests were developed for mass screening, these cutoff points are usually set quite low in order to detect as many suspicious samples as possible. This is one of the reasons there are many false positives. They might be set much higher for high-risk populations such as intravenous drug users and sexually active homosexuals, and if set too high, they might produce many false negatives (indications that the person tested does *not* carry the virus when actually he or she does).

The Western Blot test also uses virus grown in the the laboratory. This is separated by electrical currents into its component proteins in a gel and then transferred ("blotted") onto special paper. The blood sample is added, and antibodies that attach ("bind") to the viral proteins can be detected by methods using radioactivity. These show up when the paper is exposed to X-ray film in the form of bands ("hot spots") indicating the presence of antibody. (In some tests, instead of using radioactivity, the antibodies may be detected using an enzyme. In this case a colour reaction occurs in the presence of the antibody-enzyme complex.) The Western Blot test also requires interpretation of its results, for example in determining visually when a band is present, and in deciding which bands indicate the presence of AIDS antibody. Other complications, too, may arise: If the virus preparation used in the test is contaminated (for example, with antigens from the cells in which it was grown), it may produce a false result. Occasionally, despite the fact there may be no virus present in the preparation, the test may indicate that there is; this is called "non-specific binding," and can mislead the person who interprets the test. The virus preparation is bought from commercial sources, and cases have occurred in which whole batches have been unusable.

How false findings can occur

Most of us have probably been used to thinking of medical tests as showing whether we have or have not got such and such a disease. We can see from how the AIDS tests work how much more complex the picture is. False positive results with these tests may occur for a variety of reasons, some of which are simply not known. Other reasons may be the biological variations inherent in individuals. Still other variations may occur because of subjective bias in the evaluator. False *negatives* may likewise be simply due to biologic variation, or they may occur in individuals who produce lower-than-average levels of antibody or none at all.

As example of a false positive a young infant born to a mother who tests positive, may show positive because of antibodies the infant has temporarily acquired from the mother, although the infant itself may not be infected. On the other hand, infants actually infected with HIV may not develop antibodies for a long time.

All of this means that behind the many proposals that have been made for mass AIDS testing of whole populations, for screening of special groups of people such as immigrants, applicants for life insurance, or students and teachers in private schools and so on, lies a false premise. These tests were not — and cannot be — designed to do such tasks. Furthermore, when we examine the effects AIDS testing can have on individuals, it is easy to see why the subject is so contentious. It is plain. too, how important it is that the test results should be interpreted to the individuals on whom they are carried out.

Why test?

In considering under what circumstances testing should be carried out, the first question that needs to be answered is, ''What do we expect to accomplish by doing so?'' It is obvious that there should be very good reasons for carrying out AIDS tests under any circumstances. There are three main reasons for testing, all aimed at controlling the disease:

1. To gain information about the incidence of the disease that will help us to understand how it spreads and thus to limit it.

2. To provide information to people who are tested that will change or reinforce their behaviour in such a way as to limit spread.

3. To identify HIV-infected individuals so as to limit the spread of the virus, as in blood- and organ-donation programs.

From what has been said about the imperfections and uncertainties of the AIDS tests, and because high-risk individuals are unlikely to volunteer for mandatory testing, it is clear that mandatory mass testing of the entire population would not provide accurate statistical information about the infection to epidemiologists (quite apart from the cost involved, which would be considerable at $4 for a ELISA and $120 for a Western Blot test). What is more, one-time testing would be useless because any person found non-infected one day might easily become infected the next. Repeated testing would be required, which is obviously not feasible with a whole population.

If we are not going to test everybody, then whom are we going to test? Will the people to be tested agree voluntarily, or will they have to be coerced or compelled? Should their test results be available to others as well as themselves — and if so, to whom? Should individuals who ask for tests be assured of anonymity? If we decide voluntary testing is best for most people, are there special cases in which mandatory testing might be necessary? These are the kinds of questions that have to be answered concerning this complex question. Let's look at them.

Who should be tested?

The considered opinion of the Royal Society of Canada's Committee on AIDS, after much deliberation, is that the best approach that can be made in Canada, under current conditions, is to use testing judiciously on a voluntary and an anonymous or confidential basis. Every Canadian should have access to AIDS tests, but because of the potentially damaging effects of a positive result, such a test should only be administered after counselling to make sure the person being tested fully understands the implications. Furthermore, counselling should be offered one more time to such persons *after* test results are revealed to them. And finally the results should be anonymous or confidential.

The reasons for this are that severe psychological and social reactions may follow a positive AIDS test. Even if honest attempts are made to keep the results confidential, absolute confidentiality cannot be guaranteed because of the near-hysterical climate of opinion in which we currently find ourselves concerning this disease. The case of the Nova Scotia teacher referred to in the Introduction was one in which the doctor who ordered the test kept the result confidential — but one of his employees didn't. In this kind of climate, if others know that an individual has even undergone HIV testing, regardless of the result, then serious consequences could follow.

For such reasons, each person contemplating asking for a test should carefully consider the advisability of doing so, and perhaps discuss why he or she thinks a test would be advisable with a family physician or a staff member of an AIDS counselling clinic (the Royal Society committee urges that such clinics be widely available across Canada). Those considering taking the test will usually have reason to think they may somehow have become exposed to the AIDS virus. A discussion with an informed AIDS professional could set these fears to rest.

Those who wish to be tested may include persons who have received blood transfusions before the blood supply was screened for HIV (i.e. before November, 1985), or those who have received sperm, or tissue or organ transplants, before screening was carried out. Those who have been sexual partners or who have shared needles with such recipients may also wish to be tested, as might men or women who have had many sexual partners whom they suspect might belong to high-risk groups. Others desirous of testing may include health-care workers who have been exposed to body fluids of an infected person, and persons seeking health care whose symptoms suggest HIV infection as a possible factor in their illness.

The true willingness of some persons in so-called voluntary testing situations may be questioned; for example, testing children as a condition of adoption or admission to school, day-care, foster homes or custodial institutions, is unlikely to be truly voluntary and would put the children in an invidious position. The same could be said for testing as a condition of employment.

Voluntary or mandatory testing?

Rather than testing the population as a whole, and in order to have a better evaluation of the epidemic, the Royal Society committee believes that selected segments of the population should be tested, and as soon as possible. Useful information about the prevalence of the disease could be gained in this way. The most useful information would come from groups at high relative risk from the disease, such as homosexual men, intravenous drug users, prostitutes and prison inmates. How strongly such testing should be encouraged for an individual should be based on the particular risk group to which the individual belongs, the type of risk behaviour in which he or she is involved, the likelihood that the individual could infect others, and the likelihood that the test finding would influence his or her behaviour. This brings up the question of whether the tests should be voluntary or mandatory.

The only cases in which mandatory testing is recommended by the committee are among donors of blood, sperm and ova, body organs and tissues, or breast milk. The reason is that the greatest possible effort must be made to prevent the virus being spread, which would almost certainly happen if such donors were infected (although in the case of breast milk, passage of the virus has not been proved). Identification is necessary to prevent infected people from becoming donors. In the case of donors for artificial insemination, testing is recommended at the time of donation, after which the sperm should be frozen and the donor tested again in six months' time. If the donor's blood test is still negative then, the frozen sperm may be used.

Apart from these cases, testing should always be carried out on a voluntary and confidential basis, the committee recommends. Testing involves competing interests, each of which is valid, but which cannot always be reconciled. Persons who are to be tested have legitimate interests in privacy and in the freedom to make autonomous decisions about their own bodies. Their interests must be weighed against the possibly conflicting rights of others. The general principle to follow is that individual rights should be respected and preferred to restrictive measures perceived to be for the protection of society as a whole. When the threat to society — even perhaps to its very existence — is real and imminent, as for example in times of war, the rights of the individual may have to yield to the interests of society. The greater the risk to the public and the larger the proportion of the public at risk, the greater is the justification for interfering with individual liberty; conversely, the smaller the risk, the smaller the justification.

Legal responsibilities

Legally, decisions about mandatory testing in Canada are the responsibility of the provinces, unless AIDS is considered to have created such a national emergency that the federal parliament could pass extraordinary public-health legislation under its power of preserving peace, order and good government. (Such extraordinary legislation in any case would have to have a rational basis.) A distinction should be drawn between "mandatory testing" and "compulsory testing." Mandatory testing means testing that is obligatory under certain circumstances; for example, mandatory testing for immigrants means they must submit to testing if they want to get into the country. Compulsory testing, on the other hand, is testing that is inescapable. Current legislation does not authorize mandatory testing of everyone. Compulsory testing would affect several rights and freedoms guaranteed constitutionally by the Canadian Charter of Rights and Freedoms. A compulsory blood test might also temporarily affect an individual's right to liberty and security of person, and could involve a search or seizure.

All in all, it seems doubtful that universal mandatory testing could be justified legally, apart from the fact that such a program would be unlikely to be complied with and impossible to enforce. Experience shows that those individuals at highest risk find ways to avoid being tested. Therefore, a probable result of such a program, in the eyes of the Royal Society's legal experts, would be that "a new social system for evasion would be created, along with counterfeit certificates and a supply system." This would have important consequences. The very people who most need testing and counselling, and among whom education is most needed about how to avoid further spread of the disease, would be most likely to be missed. This would result in falsely low estimates of HIV-positives in the population, which not only would make the program scientifically invalid but would provide a false sense of security.

How about immigrants?
The question of whether immigrants should be tested has been widely debated. The United States now requires such testing. Some Canadians think this would be an appropriate procedure for Canada, since permission to settle in this country is a privilege, not a right, and since Canadian taxpayers' dollars would have to be spent to care for immigrants who fell ill with AIDS. These opinions are strengthened by the belief (whether accurate or not) that the disease was brought into Canada from a foreign country in the first place. A decision to require

HIV tests of all immigrants would be within the power of Canada's parliament. Potential immigrants are not protected by the country's human-rights legislation. Testing immigrants *already in Canada*, however, would raise an ethical question: what would we do with those found positive? Deport them? If so, what kind of medical treatment would they receive elsewhere? And where would that leave us legally, when people in Canada are entitled to the protection of Canadian law?

The closer we look at the question, the less sensible mandatory testing of immigrants seems. As we have seen, the AIDS tests are not entirely reliable, particularly with low-risk groups. AIDS is spread by voluntary behaviours, and to reject an immigrant on the basis of a blood test is to base a decision on theoretical, prospective presumed harm unrelated to the individual applicant. But the most compelling argument against it is that, in terms of preventing spread of the disease, it wouldn't really do any good; the AIDS epidemic is already well-established in Canada (which has the seventh highest reported number of cases in the world), and there are only about 80,000 immigrants to Canada every year, while there are *65 million* border crossings a year. So unless we are prepared to test every visitor on each and every visit — including, of course, our next-door neighbours, the Americans — the immigrant effort hardly seems worthwhile. This is quite apart from the fact that thousands of Canadians also come and go each year, some of whom may well pick up an HIV infection in the process.

One further aspect: exclusion of HIV-positive immigrants could work enormous hardship in certain cases. If, for example, one or more members of a family already settled in Canada were to be excluded on the basis of a blood test, it could mean keeping the family apart forever, since those once infected with the virus seem likely to remain infected for life. Whether this can be justified in human terms, on the basis of current knowledge about the disease, bears thinking about.

One suggestion that has been made is that it might be politically acceptable to test incoming immigrants and allow HIV-positives into the country provided they were kept track of once here. This presents certain difficulties. Once in the country, immigrants have the same rights as other Canadians. Moreover, it is difficult enough for an immigrant to adjust to a new society and perhaps a new language, possibly to be separated from family and to feel the inevitable discrimination suffered by a newcomer, without the state stigmatizing him or her as the carrier of a much-feared virus.

Testing for other reasons

Mandatory AIDS testing has been proposed, and in some cases enforced, in a number of other areas in Canada. One, as mentioned earlier, is for admission to certain private schools. The logic involved is difficult to understand.

The given reason is that a school has a duty to protect all its students, and that if, for example, one of these should be admitted from a country where AIDS is endemic, he or she might put fellow students at risk. Since AIDS is passed only through sexual intercourse, intravenous drug use or blood transfusion, it is hard to see how even the extremely unlikely presence of an AIDS-infected student would pose a problem, unless of course such practices were common at the school. In that case, perhaps the solution might lie elsewhere than with blood testing.

Of course, the *real* reason may be quite different. Is it possible that AIDS testing in schools may be a way of avoiding hiring a teacher who is homosexual, on the ground that such a teacher would be unlikely to risk taking an AIDS test?

Testing is now required for prospective policyholders by insurance companies, who fear quite naturally that if a sufficient number of these were to fall ill with AIDS, it might seriously deplete the companies' financial resources. Once again, the question is, what will the AIDS test tell them? With the potential for false positives and negatives that exists in such testing, is the threat of harm to individual rights justified? This seems doubtful. Some Canadian insurance companies are currently sending blood samples to the United States for AIDS testing. It is not known whether positive ELISA tests are being confirmed by Western Blot tests there, or whether policy applications are being denied simply on the basis of the ELISA tests. As we have seen, the latter would be inappropriate. And even if the ELISA test were followed by a Western Blot test, the testing circumstances in the United States can be much less rigorous and standardized than in Canada; many small commercial laboratories can be involved, and they may be using insufficiently standardized kits for this purpose. Thus even the two tests used serially could produce doubtful or even false results. Yet if an applicant were denied a policy on this basis, the rejection could become known and the results to the individual could be disastrous.

One further danger exists: in the United States, a number of insurance companies have refused policies to applicants who had already been HIV-tested before applying for a policy — and the refusal was made *regardless of whether the test had shown them to be HIV-positive or HIV-negative*. Apparently they were considered high-risk individuals simply by virtue of having been tested. Some victims of such discrimination have sought recourse through litigation.

The core of the issue

In one respect, the AIDS testing issue is like elementary particle physics — the deeper you go into it, the more complicated it gets! One thing is certain: there has been much oversimplification of the issue by those who are looking for easy answers to the AIDS problem. The fact is that there *are no easy answers*, and the result of a test alone, in the absence of any other clinical information, cannot be used blindly to indicate whether a given individual is infected by the AIDS virus. It is only circumstantial evidence.

For purposes of epidemiology — tracking the spread of the disease — the situation is quite different. Here we are looking for changes in disease prevalence and for rates of change. In such a situation, a few false results don't matter; they can be taken into account in our calculations. As indicators of how the disease is progressing, therefore, if anonymity is assured, AIDS tests are harmless and invaluable.

CHAPTER FOUR

Could Aids Transform Canadian Society?

"AIDS is different because its social effects are unparalleled in human history. It compels a reassessment of attitudes to many social phenomena, both for individuals and society as a whole. We will never look at sex, sexuality, drug misuse, death, disease or disablement in the same light. AIDS has become the hook on which to hang the paranoias of late twentieth century life."

Society Services Committee
House of Commons, UK

Despite the fact that the incidence and death rate of AIDS are currently much lower than those of many other diseases, and its threat to individuals is small compared to many other risks, AIDS could still bring about fundamental changes to Canadian society.

The reason is, as the quotation above points out, that AIDS is different from other diseases. First of all, it is a disease that primarily affects the young and those in the prime of life. Its capacity for damage, not just to individuals but also to a nation as a whole, is therefore greater; in developing countries, where it affects predominantly the better educated, it has the potential to virtually destroy any hope for the future. In some developed countries, it has already cut deeply into the pool of creative talent in theatre and the arts, and may yet carve a much wider swath. AIDS is different also because its incubation period is so long: infected persons may not produce antibody for a year or more, and may be symptom-free for as long as nine years after infection. During this time, however, they may be capable of infecting others, and so may spread the disease unwittingly.

Recently a group called the British Association for Counselling (BAC), which helps people deal with their problems through verbal interaction between counsellor and client, tried to explain what it is that makes people regard AIDS with such intensity of feeling. Its panel concluded that AIDS brings together a whole range of conditions and situations that arouse great anxiety in nearly everyone, even when encountered singly. These include the following:

The dying: We tend to avoid people who are dying because they cause us embarrassment, fear and other strong emotions.

The dead: For most of us, even viewing a dead body is stressful, and we avoid it.

The disfigured: We avoid them, perhaps even hide them away.

The disabled: Despite great efforts made recently, we still surround them with taboos.

The lonely: We tend to avoid those living alone.

Sexual minorities: Homosexuals, bisexuals, transsexuals and others are regarded with suspicion, fear and dislike.

People with sexually transmitted disease: We set up clinics to treat them anonymously and as inconspicuously as possible, illustrating our embarrassment as a society with these diseases — and perhaps with sexuality.

Drug misusers: The stereotype of the addict is one of antisocial degeneracy, despite the fact that many drugs are now accepted socially by some sectors of society.

A pronounced social stigma is attached to each of these groups, said the BAC. Think what the effect would be if all their attributes were combined in one person! Yet a person with AIDS might well belong to all — and he or she might in addition be non-European (read non-Canadian).

It is for such reasons that the AIDS epidemic is bound to have profound effects on Canadian life, by raising social, legal and ethical issues never before encountered. If we are not forewarned of these, and if we do not consider in advance what our attitudes should be to them, the epidemic could transform Canadian society in ways that run counter to our traditional values. We could even create a body of social "lepers" who will lose the rights and freedoms we have fought so hard to ensure for all.

The groups of people described above may seem outside the day-today experience of most of us (perhaps partly because we tend to avoid them). But AIDS can strike much closer to home, affecting the kinds of people we know — those who are friends, even those who live next door. When that happens, the impact of the disease hits hard. Consider, for example, the story of Louise and Paul Cranford and their family.

A case study
Louise and Paul Cranford have been married for six years. They have three children, Peter, 5, Jane, 3, Emilie, four months. (All names have been changed.) Emilie had been ill since her birth and was hospitalized for treatment of an overwhelming systemic infection. It was at this stage that the pediatrician looking after Emilie, Dr. Stark, ordered an HIV-antibody test. It was found to be positive. These results were supported by confirmatory testing. This test, together with Emilie's rapidly deteriorating state of health, enabled Dr. Stark, in consultation with other physicians, to come to a diagnosis of AIDS.

Dr. Stark arranged to meet with Paul and Louise to discuss Emilie's condition. At this time, he disclosed to them that she had AIDS, that it was extremely unlikely that she would live more than two years, and that it was very likely that she would be seriously ill throughout this time. They, of course, were devastated by this information. Probably the most devastating situation that persons can face is to be told that their child has a fatal illness. Paul and Louise were not only facing this situation, but also all the other implications and consequences of a diagnosis of AIDS.

There was no readily apparent reason why Paul or Louise should be infected with HIV, as neither of them had ever received a blood transfusion and, as far as either of them knew with respect to the other, neither of them had engaged in conduct that was risk-taking with respect to the transmission of HIV.

In fact, both of them *had* engaged in such conduct. Paul was bisexual and had had several "anonymous" homosexual encounters in gay bathhouses when he had been away on business trips. Paul's latest homosexual encounter had been in a gay bathhouse in New York 18 months previously, when he had engaged in unprotected anal intercourse. For a short time in 1980, prior to her marriage, Louise had spent six months in New York after the breakup of a long-term, live-in relationship in Toronto. During this time, she had had many male sexual partners and on two occasions had experimented with intravenous drugs, when she had shared injection equipment.

Dr. Stark suggested that both Paul and Louise and their other two children, Peter and Jane, be tested for HIV-antibody positivity. The results were that Paul and Louise were positive and the other two children were negative. It is likely, although not certain, that Louise was antibody negative at the time she gave birth to her first two children, and that she become antibody positive subsequent to that time. The only way in which this could have happened was that Paul became infected through his homosexual encounter in New York eighteen months previously and subsequently infected Louise.

Three months after his homosexual encounter in New York, Paul had gone to see his doctor in Toronto and told him that he was concerned about his recent risk-taking activities with respect to HIV transmission and that he was deeply concerned that he might have been infected. The physician, Dr. Black, explained to Paul about the availability of the HIV-antibody test, but neither encouraged nor discouraged Paul from having it. Dr. Black knew Paul was married and had two children, but had never met Louise. He did not know, because Paul did not tell him, that Paul and Louise had at that time discussed the possibility of having another baby. They had not come to any firm conclusion in this respect, although Paul knew that Louise was going to have a "three-month rest" from taking the contraceptive pill.

When Louise felt she could no longer cope psychologically with the situation that had developed after Emilie's diagnosis, she went to see her doctor to ask for a certificate for sick leave from her job. Louise presented this certificate to her employer, who asked her what had happened. Louise, in a state of great distress, explained about the baby and about her own and Paul's HIV-antibody positivity. Three days later, Louise received a registered letter, which told her that her employment was terminated and said that she would receive three months' salary in lieu of notice. Word spread around the neighbourhood that the baby and the Cranford family "had AIDS," and the principal at the school where 5-year-old Peter was in Grade 1 asked that the child be withdrawn. Likewise, the day-care centre where 3-year-old Jane stayed while both Paul and Louise worked, also refused to accept the child any longer.

Louise's employer had told one of Louise's workmates that Louise's baby, Emilie, had AIDS and that Louise was antibody positive. The workmate had children at the same school as Louise's child Peter and informed the principal. Parents of other children at the school, who also had children in the day-care centre, learned of Peter's exclusion and informed the day-care centre.

Paul, at this time, was manifesting neurological symptoms possibly attributable to HIV infection. The physician immunologist caring for him asked a neurologist colleague for a consultation, and she ordered a brain scan using nuclear magnetic resonance imaging (NMRI). However, the nuclear medicine specialists at the only hospital that had an NMR scanner refused to accept Paul or any AIDS patients because of fear of contaminating the NMRI examination chamber with HIV.

The fact that Paul had engaged in sexual activity outside his marriage was news to Louise, and she found it extremely difficult to cope with emotionally, especially because of its homosexual nature. Louise and Paul now also face a constant, ineradicable threat to their own lives and must deal with the possibility that both of them could die from AIDS and leave their other two children without parents. Paul is self-employed and has inadequate sickness and disability insurance and no life insurance, and they are not independently wealthy. This means they will not be able to provide for their own future care and that of their other two children, and must live with this knowledge and the fear and despair it produces. Paul and Louise and all their children are likely to be subject to further discrimination and stigmatization, because it has become known in their community that members of their family are infected with HIV. Whether, and if so how, to disclose the information regarding their HIV infection to their wider family, and coping with their reactions and suffering, is also a serious problem. There is also a great deal of uncertainty in this situation, especially regarding the likelihood of occurrence of serious consequences, and such uncertainty can be very difficult to live with psychologically.

Another frequently encountered impact of having knowledge that one is HIV-antibody positive is the necessity for change with respect to sexual behaviour. This may be required of Louise and Paul in relation to each other, even though they are both infected with HIV, because repeated exposure to the virus may cause them further damage. Such a change would also be required on the part of Paul with respect to any future homosexual encounters.*

Grappling with the implications of AIDS
The above tragic story illustrates in graphic fashion many of the potential questions and problems raised by AIDS.

• The need for widespread and easily available information on how to avoid getting the disease.

• The moral and legal obligations of husbands and wives to disclose to each other risky activities that they have undertaken, and if physicians know of these, their responsibility to consider whether to warn spouses.

• The obligation of obstetricians to offer expectant mothers HIV-antibody tests.

• Moral and legal questions surrounding discrimination in the workplace and at school.

• The need for counselling before and after HIV testing to help people cope with a positive result.

• The moral and professional justification (or lack of it) for health-care personnel refusing access to treatment to HIV-antibody positive people.

• The rights of persons with AIDS to adequate medical care if they cannot afford it personally.

Some of these are dealt with elsewhere in this book. Here we will consider problems involving privacy and discriminatory treatment to persons with AIDS, problems presented by AIDS in the workplace and among indigenous peoples, and finally, some legal implications.

Confidentiality
We have previously mentioned the case of the Nova Scotia primary-school teacher whose position became untenable as a result of a breach of privacy in the office of his physician. The story of Louise and Paul,

---

* A composite example re-created from actual cases. From *Social Consequences of AIDS,* prepared for *AIDS: Grappling With the Theological and Ethical Issues,* a bi-national (Canada/United States) consultation held in Toronto, Ontario, Canada, October 23-25, 1987, by Dr. Margaret A. Sommerville, Professor, Faculty of Law and Faculty of Medicine, McGill University, Montreal, and Director, McGill Centre for Medicine, Ethics and Law. To be published by Pilgrim Press, New York, Spring, 1988.

though quite different, provides another illustration of the serious results that can occur when private medical information becomes public. The growing use of computers to store medical records greatly increases anxieties about their confidentiality.

Recognition of the need for confidentiality in health matters goes back at least to Hippocrates in the fourth century BC and was acknowledged in the Hippocratic Oath, which includes this clause:

> Whatever, in connection with my professional practice, or not in connection with it, I see or hear, in the life of men, which ought not to be spoken abroad, I will not divulge, as reckoning that all such should be kept secret.

The Canadian Medical Association's code of ethics likewise provides that

> The ethical physician . . . will keep in confidence information derived from his patient or from a colleague, regarding a patient, and divulge it only with the permission of the patient except when the law requires him to do so . . . .

Provincial legislation in Canada reinforces these admonitions. In Ontario, the Health Disciplines Act says that "professional misconduct on the part of a physician includes revealing patient information to any person other than the patient without the patient's consent, unless required to do so by law." Quebec has comparable legislation.

Physicians are not the only health-care workers whose treatment of confidential information is regulated. Nor are they the only people in health care who may work with HIV-antibody positive people, or learn that an individual is seropositive (i.e. whose blood has tested positive for HIV). But sometimes the rules under which they operate are ambiguous insofar as AIDS is concerned. For example, dentists in Ontario are required to keep confidential information *concerning the patient's dental condition.* But what if the dentist finds that a patient is HIV-infected? Is he prohibited from passing on *that* information?

Nurses may learn early of a patient's HIV infection. A school nurse or a nurse in a corporation may be given such information in confidence: Is she required to give that information to her employer? Others who may become privy to such information are pharmacists, psychiatrists, psychologists or counsellors. The need for them to respect the privacy of the information is as apparent as it is in the case of physicians.

As noted, physicians are adjured to maintain medical records as confidential except where required by law to reveal them. AIDS *must* by law be reported to provincial health authorities in every province in Canada and in the two territories, but the manner of reporting required varies. Thus Alberta, British Columbia, Manitoba, New Brunswick and Newfoundland require that reporting include the name and address of the infected person, while Quebec specifically prohibits reporting of the person's name and designates him or her by a number, age, sex and municipality only.

Factors involved in choosing reporting methods
Which method of reporting is preferable? To decide, we should consider why reporting is done. One reason is to protect society from further spread of the disease. This involves knowing how widely the disease has already spread. Such epidemiological information can quite satisfactorily be supplied without the names of infected individuals being involved. If preventing spread of the disease were to involve isolation and treatment of those infected, identifying the infected persons might serve a purpose. But there is no effective treatment for AIDS, and it is obviously impractical to isolate 30,000 or more individuals, so such identification seems pointless. If, besides being pointless, identification would expose persons with AIDS to great social risks, it seems not only clearly undesirable but morally unacceptable, and anonymous reporting appears to be the preferable method.

Non-infected individuals in society also have an interest in what risks they may run in respect to communicable, fatal diseases. But identifying persons with AIDS by name to health authorities will scarcely reduce these risks, because, as we have seen, the disease is not spread by casual contact, and every individual must be personally responsible for the risks he or she runs in sexual contacts.

A special problem might arise if a doctor found himself or herself knowing that a patient was HIV-infected and faced with the problem of whether or not to tell a spouse or sexual partner. Could the physician be found guilty of professional misconduct for doing so? In an analogous case, a physician who warned an intended victim of the possibility that one of his patients might do the victim violence was found *not guilty* of professional misconduct, despite the fact that the circumstances of the charge had been established.

But in the case of AIDS, revealing such information to a spouse or sexual partner might not do any good, because the partner might already be infected. And in some cases the partner might have become infected from someone else. For such reasons it does not seem justified to make the reporting of patient information to a partner compulsory.

Special cases

But what should be done about an individual — male or female — known to be HIV-infected, who states openly that he or she intends to go on having sexual relations despite the risk to others? Such incidents have been known to occur. At an AIDS symposium of the American Association for the Advancement of Science in Boston in February, 1988, Gordon R. Hough, a staff member at the Bailey House AIDS Resource in New York City, commented: "I personally know three people who are HIV-infected who say they are going to take as many people as possible with them." It would seem only sensible to pass legislation that permits a health-care provider to disclose such information to those in danger without consent of the patient.

There have also been questions raised about how to deal with irresponsible individuals, such as the Vanier, Ontario, man who donated blood to the Red Cross while knowing that he was HIV-infected. Screening picked up his contaminated blood immediately after it was donated in October, 1987. To protect society, quarantine or some sort of compulsory isolation has been proposed for such individuals. Because of the complexities involved, it would seem advisable to deal with this sort of case on an individual basis.

Discrimination

As we have seen, some persons with AIDS and those who have tested HIV-positive have already suffered discrimination in Canada. Besides those already mentioned, two complaints of discrimination concerning provision of services were made to the Ontario Human Rights Commission in 1986, four cases of discrimination in employment were before the board at time of writing, and four other cases were being investigated by the British Columbia Council of Human Rights.

We have seen earlier why the British Association for Counselling believes people react with strong emotions to persons with AIDS. Their reasoning helps explain why discrimination against such individuals occurs. But there is something more involved: fear of becoming infected. As we have also seen, such fears are ill-founded, because AIDS is not transmitted through casual contacts such as those that occur in the workplace or in schools. Such fear, therefore, is irrational and based on ignorance of the true situation. (In extreme cases, it takes on attributes of paranoia.)

Other factors, too, may figure in the fear of AIDS. The disease is thought of by many as a homosexual one, despite evidence to the contrary. And because some condemn homosexuality, AIDS is seen by them as a judgment from God brought to bear on "evil" homosexuals. Patrick Buchanan, columnist for the *New York Post* and a former speechwriter for U.S. President Ronald Reagan, wrote in 1983: "The poor homosexuals — they have declared war upon Nature, and now Nature is exacting an awful retribution." To such people, this belief may justify feelings of antipathy, and thus discrimination, not only against persons with AIDS but against all homosexuals.

Commented Allan M. Brandt in *Law, Medicine & Health Care*, the journal of the American Society of Law and Medicine: "In this context, homosexuality — not a virus — *causes* AIDS. Therefore, homosexuality itself is feared as if it were a communicable, lethal disease. After a generation of work to have homosexuality removed as a disease from the psychiatric diagnostic manuals, it had suddenly reappeared as an infectious, terminal disease."

A similar line of thought may lie behind discrimination against certain ethnic or racial groups, such as Africans. As noted in Chapter One, AIDS is believed by some scientists to have originated in Africa, though they can only speculate how this might have happened. This belief has fuelled the fears of those who mistrust Africans and also believe them to have bizarre sexual customs and has led to a conviction — totally unfounded — that "Africans are responsible for the AIDS epidemic" and therefore should be shunned.* Finally, there are the intravenous drug users who contract AIDS. Such people are thought by many to be "lost souls" who exist on the fringes of society, who have no willpower

---

* A recent Reuters news story said researchers reported from the South American port of Belém that they had found antibodies to an AIDS-like virus in 100 Indians living in the Amazon jungle, reviving the monkey — transfer theory but deflecting suspicions about Africans.

and who are antisocial. There is therefore little sympathy for them, and discrimination against them is made easy.

The basic fallacy underlying discrimination seems to be a belief that, somehow, discriminatory actions will help or protect those who promote or practise them. They will do nothing of the kind. But what they will *certainly* do is harm those discriminated against. Discriminatory treatment based on prejudice runs counter to the basic tenets of Canadian society; it offends public policy and cannot be justified. Morality, ethics, law and humanitarian impulses are all opposed to it. Even those religions and value systems in which homosexuality and drug abuse are morally unacceptable should condemn the "sin" and not the "sinner." The fight against the spread of AIDS will be won only by persuading those who behave unwisely to change, not by discriminating against them. Ultimately, discrimination will backfire and harm the discriminator, because it will not work, and unless dangerous behaviour is curbed, the disease will continue to spread.

AIDS in the workplace

Two groups of people are concerned about the presence of AIDS in the workplace: those who are infected and those who fear becoming infected. Those infected want to avoid being discriminated against, and those who are ill with AIDS want their needs as people with a disease accommodated. Those who fear becoming infected are chiefly concerned that they do not contract the disease.

We have dealt with the discrimination issue above. But beyond this, persons with AIDS or HIV infection need to be accepted by their colleagues and not ostracized. Workers who fear the possibility of infection need reassurance — based on scientific findings and experience with the disease — that they are not dangerously exposed by the presence of infected fellow workers. But that may not be enough, because they know that the record of employers in occupational disease is less than exemplary, and they will be aware of many examples of misinformation on hazards having been supplied by employers, or simply of lack of information.

The experience of the asbestos industry is far from reassuring in this respect. So is that of Black Lung disease in mines. Observers 100 years ago had noted the high incidence of upper respiratory disease among miners, but their condition was ascribed to something called deprecatingly "miners' asthma," or to emotional disorder or even malingering. It was not until 1978 that legislation was amended to help those whose health had been impaired by long years of employment in the mines. No new facts brought this about — just a new judgment about the facts.

So employees may be reluctant to accept employers' assurances that AIDS does not create a risk for them. One solution is to develop educational programs tailored to the conditions of each workplace. It should draw on the extensive medical and epidemiological material showing that AIDS is not transmitted by casual contact, such as the studies of health-care workers referred to in Chapter One. Such a program should be designed co-operatively by management, unions and employees together with occupational health and safety representatives. And education should consist not only of scientific information but also of initiatives designed to promote tolerance of employees with AIDS and support for them.

For those whose workplace is part of the health-care system, special steps are needed. We cannot assume that doctors and nurses, because of their special training, are necessarily well informed about AIDS. Educational sessions should be arranged for all health-care workers and attendance required on a periodic basis to ensure they remain well-informed. Informative published material, such as the Ontario Ministry of Health's publication *Understanding AIDS and HIV Infection: Information for Hospitals and Health Professionals,* is already available and should be used.

Nor can we assume that because health-care professionals are highly educated they will necessarily be tolerant and caring with respect to AIDS patients. A study of the attitudes of randomly selected physicians in three large cities in three different states of the U.S. found that "the AIDS diagnosis carried emotional charge and elicits judgmental, negative evaluations about the patient even by health-care providers." Such attitudes can interfere with a doctor-patient relationship. The physician's job is to counsel, educate, treat, heal and support the sick, not to judge them. Persons with AIDS and those who are HIV-positive need a trusting relationship with doctors if the doctors are to treat them and help control the spread of HIV infection.

Delicate ethical issues arise in relationships between AIDS patients and their doctors. For example, there may be a great reluctance to discuss the patient's wishes about death, and when patients have not expressed such wishes in advance, hospital staff may be forced to make decisions on the spot about heroic means of supporting life. Such issues will be discussed in the next chapter.

Special problems of indigenous peoples
Inuit and Indian people may appear to be at greater risk of AIDS than many other Canadians for a number of reasons. One is that many of them live in isolated communities where they might be thought to lack information about the disease. Many are also believed to suffer a feeling of powerlessness to bring about changes in their lives, although this is changing for some as they gain more control of their institutions. Thirdly, for whatever reason, the rate of at least one sexually transmitted disease in such populations is higher than in others in Canada (in 1985, the rate of reported cases of gonorrhea in the Northwest Territories was 2,371.3 per 100,000, compared with 38.5 in Prince Edward Island — the lowest provincial rate — and 297.8 in Manitoba — the highest. In the Yukon, the rate was 837.7). And, as stated in Chapter One, the incidence of AIDS is higher among people with a history of other sexually transmitted diseases.

Historically, numerous examples can be found of native peoples being decimated by new diseases. In *Plagues and Peoples,* history professor William H. McNeill attributes the Spanish conquest of Mexico to the ravages of a smallpox epidemic. The Spaniards had some immunity from previous contact with the disease, but the Aztecs did not. The combined physical and psychological effects of the epidemic, says McNeill, allowed Hernando Cortez, starting off with fewer than 600 men, to conquer an Aztec empire with millions of subjects.

In the case of AIDS, of course, it is not just the native population that has no immunity — it is all of us. But their susceptibility to infection may be higher. We must, however, be careful how we regard the reasons for this, if we are to avoid the kind of scapegoating mentioned earlier. For example, it is a common belief among Canadians who are not themselves Inuit, that visitors in Inuit society have sexual access to the wives of their hosts. Anthropologists tell us this is not the case; a form of co-spouse relationships did exist among the Inuit that was mostly but not exclusively polygamous, but this was fenced about with elaborate rules and regulations. Rather than accept such common travellers' tales, those involved in policymaking or educational programs must base their proposals on reliable and sound information about the sexual practices of Canada's diverse cultural groups — and this calls for research (see Chapters Five and Six).

Those who work in Northern Canada point out that one reason sexually transmitted disease rates are higher in the North than elsewhere in the country is that the reporting system is better. They admit that there is a relatively high rate of sexual activity there, but note that this may at least partly be due to the fact that a high proportion of the population consists of young people.

"Our concern here," says Dr. David Kinloch, regional Medical Officer of Health for the Northwest Territories in Yellowknife, "is that the potential for spread is obviously greater (among a small, isolated population), even if the risk of AIDS getting into the community is low. That's why we're emphasizing keeping it out."

Nancy Williamson, public-health nurse in Yellowknife, disagrees with the idea that Northerners may have less information about AIDS than people further south. She says that the NWT have one of the most progressive AIDS programs in the country, with posters in 10 languages, as well as pamphlets, tapes and videos. In March, 1988, television spot announcements were due to appear, also in 10 languages.

Dr. Kinloch suggests that precisely because Northern communities are smaller and remote, they may offer an opportunity to set an example in AIDS prevention programs, and thus lead the country in this regard.

Provincial legislation

Most discrimination that may be suffered by persons with AIDS or those who are seropositive — for example, with respect to goods and services, accommodation and employment — is governed by provincial human-rights codes. However, this legislation varies in both language and intent from province to province. Because of the uncertainties that might occur as a result, it seems desirable that all human-rights legislation in Canada should be amended to prohibit discrimination based on HIV seropositivity or infection — and even on *beliefs* that individuals are HIV seropositive or infected. Both policymakers and the public should also be made aware through educational programs of what the human-rights codes say about such matters.

Provincial public-health legislation already covers an enormous array of powers. These were passed at different times in history to deal with specific disease problems, and they reflect the social values of their times. With a disease such as AIDS, any legislative attempts to control the disease must be carefully evaluated. It must be recognized that while legislation can help to control a disease, it cannot *by itself* control it. For example, many provinces have laws requiring individuals who believe themselves to be infected to seek medical treatment. If the idea behind this legislation is to reduce the spread of disease through treatment, how does it apply to a disease for which no effective treatment exists?

Repressive legislation

Because of the strong views that AIDS elicits, there is a danger that some who hold such views may attempt to have repressive legislation passed. For example, William F. Buckley, Jr., the conservative U.S. writer, put forward in the *New York Times* in 1986 the position of "those whose anxiety to protect the public impels them to give subordinate attention to the civil amenities of those who suffer from AIDS and primary attention to the safety of those who do not." Logically, he suggested, this leads to the proposal that everyone "detected with AIDS should be tattooed in the upper forearm, to protect common needle users, and on the buttocks, to protect the victimization of other homosexuals."

In Canada, a medical officer of health in 1988 proposed that quarantine should be considered for some AIDS carriers; in 1985, at a U.S. conference, Dr. Vernon Mark, a Harvard neurosurgeon and formerly a chief of service at Boston City Hospital, had suggested quarantining AIDS-virus carriers who persist in "irresponsible" behaviour, on a state-owned island in Buzzard's Bay that was once a leper colony.

Dr. Margaret A. Sommerville, director of the McGill Centre for Medicine, Ethics and Law, discussed this kind of thinking at a Canada/U.S. consultation called "AIDS: Grappling with the Theological and Ethical Issues" in October, 1987:

"The most extreme example of the latter type of intervention would be to seek to eliminate AIDS from the community by executing every person who is HIV-antibody positive or suffering from AIDS," she said.

Dr. Sommerville proposes, rather, that in making decisions about public policy for AIDS, "our analysis . . . must start from a 'prima facie' presumption of respect for all persons, including for their rights or liberties. This means that persons seeking to infringe on such rights or liberties have the obligation of justifying their interventions. Such interventions will only be justified when the benefits that they offer clearly outweight the harms; they are the least invasive, least restrictive alternatives reasonably available and are likely to be effective in achieving a justified outcome; and they are not inherently absolutely unacceptable."

Even those who are prone to adopt strict views about HIV-infected people and persons with AIDS, and who think of compassionate solutions as fit only for "bleeding hearts," should bear in mind one further factor when pondering what society should do about the AIDS problem. Legislation that intrudes too far on one's personal rights and freedoms, or is too restrictive, may produce effects the *opposite* of those desired. If HIV carriers and people with AIDS are made to feel stigmatized, discriminated against, isolated or ostracized — or like criminals — they may well begin to behave in a way they would not otherwise do — in the very way, in fact, that the repressive measures were designed to prevent. And this could result in a *greater* spread of AIDS than would have been the case if they had been compassionately and humanely treated. After all, a person who faces an early death might say: "What have I got to lose?" In the end, in such a situation, all of us would be the losers.

Many people in Canada today seem to feel that when something is wrong, all we have to do to remedy the situation is pass a law. Thoughtful jurists tell us this is not the case, and in fact the opposite might be true: passing a law might actually make things worse. If we can accomplish the same end *without* passing a law, we may all be better off.

Finally, the kinds of conclusions we come to concerning AIDS will have an importance far beyond the disease situation itself. As Dr. Somerville points out, "Decisions taken in the AIDS context will affect [the ethical and legal tone of the society] both directly and more indirectly through their precedent-setting effect far outside the 'AIDS arena.'"

CHAPTER FIVE

The Price To Pay

The costs Canadians will have to pay for the care and treatment of persons with AIDS and those infected with HIV are high. Obviously, the more Canadians there are in these categories, the higher the costs will be, so in addition to humanitarian reasons there is a strong economic incentive to prevent further spread of the disease. Prevention, too, will be expensive.

The increased burden on the Canadian health-care system resulting from AIDS comes at a time when higher costs are already growing as a result of the greater proportion of older people in the population, who traditionally require more services than do the young.

The costs involved can be divided into direct and indirect costs, and further into personal and non-personal costs. Direct costs are those incurred in the treatment and prevention of AIDS and HIV infections. Indirect costs represent the loss to society of an individual's productive capacity resulting from illness or death. Personal costs include all those costs involved in providing continuing health care, while non-personal costs are those involved in screening, counselling, education, administration and research.

In 1987, an estimated $75 million was the personal direct cost incurred in the treatment of HIV-infected individuals in Canada. This figure includes in-patient and out-patient care, drugs, home care and physicians' payments. Non-personal costs for the same period are estimated at another $54 million at least. This will bring the total of all direct costs to at least $129 million for the year — and they might go as high as $200 million.

The total indirect costs for the same period — what the country lost in productivity — are estimated at between $150 million and $350 million (depending on the assumptions used), or between 0.3 percent and 0.6 percent of the country's gross national product.

If we use the higher of the two figures for indirect costs, the total of direct and indirect costs comes to about *half a billion dollars* for the year. To put this figure into some perspective, consider that it costs around $80,000 to $100,000 for four years of medical school. To become a doctor, an individual needs, in addition to the years in medical school, two or three years of undergraduate university education and two or more years of clinical training. But ignoring the costs of the latter (which are too varied to estimate) we could say that the money spent on AIDS for just one year could have paid for the medical school training of between 5,000 and 6,000 doctors. Looking at it another way, the federal government in May, 1986, pledged to spend some $39 million on AIDS prevention and treatment over the following five years. What AIDS actually *cost* Canada in the following year alone amounted to about *12 times* that amount.

Individual treatment costs
On an annual basis, each person diagnosed as having AIDS costs about $82,500 to treat. In-patient hospital costs account for more than two-thirds of this. In Toronto General Hospital, the costs of caring for all AIDS patients were higher by approximately 46 percent than the reimbursement provided by the provincial health ministry. We cannot say unequivocally that it costs much more to treat AIDS patients than those with *any* other disease because the statistics are simply not available to make such a comparison. It does cost more to treat an AIDS patient than the *"average"* patient; even for the *least costly* AIDS patients, figures at Toronto General Hospital were 31 percent higher. Treating a condition such as the final stages of kidney disease can be extremely expensive: in Kingston General Hospital, with three dialyses a week, the dialysis costs alone were $20,592 annually. This means that the lifetime costs of such a condition may be much higher than the lifetime costs of HIV infections — but that is at least partly because the kidney-disease patient may live longer. Average lifetime hospital costs for AIDS patients were approximately $50,000 in Vancouver and $75,000 in Quebec.

Incidental costs
In addition to hospital costs directly attributable to AIDS patients, we must add incidental costs incurred through the use of extra precautions taken by health-care workers in laboratories, operating rooms and emergency departments. For example, many more gloves and gowns

are used when blood is drawn or analyzed, or when direct contact is possible with bodily fluids and wastes.

Several Ontario hospitals are planning to implement universal precautions so that all patients and specimens will be considered potentially infectious. This involves extra expense in terms of equipment and staff time; for example, it usually takes an average of 10-15 minutes to take a blood sample, but with extra precautions it takes 40-45 minutes. To put these precautionary plans into place will cost an estimated $500,000 at Toronto General Hospital and $250,000 at Ottawa General Hospital.

Costs of screening are increasing as more individuals are tested for HIV antibody. In Ontario and British Columbia, the number of tests performed during the first seven months of 1987, excluding those done by the Canadian Red Cross, doubled compared to the number carried out in the whole of 1986. If this is true of the rest of Canada, 150,000 tests will have been carried out in 1987 at a cost of $2.5 million, exclusive of counselling costs. If counselling took half an hour each for pre-and post-test counselling, these costs (based on Ontario physicians' charges) will have amounted to about $13 million in 1987.

Physicians' costs
AIDS patients are difficult for physicians to treat for a number of reasons, one of them being the large amount of time that must be spent in doing so. Some doctors, however, may spend *less* time than with an average patient, either because of fears of the disease or discomfort with homosexuals. Two U.S. studies found that "homophobia" and a lack of medical competence in dealing with AIDS patients was troubling: it reportedly occurred especially in rural communities. Other difficult factors are that doctors cannot bill for what may amount to considerable time giving advice on the telephone or in completing forms required for using experimental drugs.

AIDS patients may require a large number of specialists as well as a general practitioner. The best current estimate is that, if counselling is included, it may cost between $7,000 and $10,000 a year for physicians' services for an AIDS patient.

Nurses and other professionals
Many kinds of professionals play a role in the care of an HIV-infected person: social workers, psychologists, bereavement counsellors, clergy,

physiotherapists, occupational therapists, dentists and dieticians. But nursing care may be the largest single cost involved. At St. Paul's Hospital in Vancouver, the head nurses have estimated that 9.8 hours of nursing care are required every 24 hours for each AIDS patient, while only 5.2 hours are budgeted for. Preliminary results of a study underway at Montreal General and Royal Victoria Hospitals show that a person with AIDS requires three to five times more nursing care than the average hospital patient. In a 24-hour period, 15 hours are needed to care for an AIDS patient, and if admission to intensive care is involved, two nurses may devote all their time to a single patient.

Drug and screening costs

AIDS patients need expensive drugs. Costs will vary greatly from patient to patient and according to different physicians' preferences and other factors. New drugs tend to be expensive: AZT costs about $250 for 100 capsules, and a daily dose is 12 capsules. The yearly cost for this drug thus totals $10,950. The antiviral drug Acyclovir, used for herpes infections, can cost up to $200 a day for intravenous treatments, while long-term therapy will cost about $10 a day, totalling perhaps $2,000 over six months.

In Canada, the annual cost of screening blood donors to safeguard the transfusion blood supply is about $6 million. Pilot projects are being conducted to determine whether it is feasible for some patients to set aside some of their own blood in advance of the time when they will need a transfusion (this is known as autologous blood transfusion). Based on U.S. experience, such a program in Canada would cost about $6 million annually.

Children with AIDS

One of the most tragic aspects of AIDS is that it affects children as well as adults. The children contract HIV either via an infected parent or, before blood and blood products were screened and heat-treated, through blood transfusions or clotting factors. Twenty-six children in Canada have AIDS, 22 of them as a result of having a parent-at-risk. Eleven of the children have been under one year of age. There are bound to be many more if the expected second wave of the epidemic occurs in intravenous drug users.

The majority of AIDS cases among the newborn in Canada have occurred in the Montreal area; nearly all have been children of parents from areas where HIV infection is endemic. Others are hemophiliacs; 40 percent of the 120 hemophiliac children being monitored at the Hospital for Sick Children in Toronto are HIV-positive, but only one has developed AIDS. In southern Ontario, 70 percent of those being followed are HIV-positive, while in Ottawa, 60 percent are seropositive.

Ste. Justine Hospital is the major pediatric-care hospital and also the one most involved in pediatric HIV infection. By the end of 1986, 35 families were being followed, 38 of whose children were HIV-infected; of these, 16 had died, five had no symptoms and six had AIDS. The majority were under three years of age.

The sicker children required 22 hours of nursing care out of every 24, while others needed nine. Most needed 15 hours a day of nursing care. The hospital costs for these children were about 60 percent higher than those of children admitted for other reasons. It will cost an estimated $669,543 in operating costs annually for the AIDS program at the hospital in the future, based on past experience.

New York has had the greatest experience with pediatric AIDS because of the high incidence among drug users. There, children require long hospital stays because of a lack of community facilities and because their parents often cannot take care of them. Newborn babies often have to stay in hospital a long time because antibodies passed to them from their mothers take up to a year to disappear, and until it is determined whether or not the baby has HIV, it is difficult to find foster homes. If AIDS cases among drug users increase in Canada, we will face similar problems, concentrated in centres with the largest number of drug users — Vancouver, Toronto and Montreal. The financial burdens will affect most acutely the children's hospitals in these cities.

Future costs of AIDS
Future costs will, of course, increase as the number of persons with HIV infections and AIDS increases. An estimated 6,000 to 11,000 persons in Canada will have been diagnosed as having AIDS by the end of 1992. Based on the length of time individuals with AIDS now live, the total direct costs for that year could be anywhere between $165

million and $247 million, or between 1.2 percent and 2.1 percent of all health-care expenditures. The uncertainty in this prediction lies in not knowing what changes may occur in the epidemic to modify current trends.

We can calculate how much we could save in health-care system expenditures by preventing the epidemic from spreading further, however. Preventing just one person from becoming infected could save at least $82,400 annually in direct medical expenditures; it could also save the economy between $325,700 and $800,017 annually in lost productivity. If *half* of a projected 6,274 cases by 1992 were prevented, this would represent savings of well over a billion dollars.

How will we take care of people with AIDS?
The Canadian health-care system is one of the best in the world. It is also expensive to run. In 1985, the latest year for which statistics are available, $39.2 billion was spent on health care in Canada (both public and private); this constituted 8.5 percent of the country's GNP.

But already the public health-care system is strained, with shortages of both personnel and funds. Add to this the further demands that will be placed on the system by an indeterminate number of AIDS patients, and we have a problem. The system was never designed to handle such a situation. AIDS has become a large-scale, rapidly expanding, labour-intensive and socially disruptive problem.

First of all, no central administrative mechanism exists for planning and co-ordinating medical care for HIV-infected people. And it's not as though the problem is going to go away — it can only become worse. HIV infection can be controlled eventually, but as pointed out in Chapter Two, the AIDS virus will not be eliminated from the face of the earth. Controlling it will be a permanent problem. This will require effective planning and co-ordination on a national scale. There is no way this can be done at the moment.

In early 1988, in the whole of Canada, there were only 19 beds officially assigned for active treatment of AIDS patients. Yet as of May, 1988, there were 781 people with AIDS in the country and about 10 percent or 78 of these might have been expected to be in hospital on any given day. Eighteen of the AIDS beds were located in a single hospital: St. Paul's Hospital, Vancouver. Quebec, with one-third of the nation's cases, had a single bed available for AIDS terminal care, in the palliative care unit of Montreal's Royal Victoria Hospital. Despite the wide variety of health-care facilities set up for specific purposes such as cancer or arthritis, no plans yet existed to establish facilities dedicated to active treatment of AIDS patients in either Toronto or Montreal.

Most AIDS patients in Canada are concentrated in a few large teaching hospitals. Hardly any of these have admission policies developed specifically for the disease, and most have only recently begun to develop comprehensive approaches to deal with AIDS problems. At present, AIDS patients are managed within the context of policies developed for infectious diseases generally. This has meant diversion of already sharply restricted funds, space and other resources. As a result, resources are strained and doctors working with AIDS patients are greatly overworked.

Psychiatric care for the HIV-infected is almost non-existent in Canada, yet it is essential because of the extreme stress, alienation, guilt and denial involved. As noted before, many HIV-infected persons become severely depressed and some suicidal. Many also develop dementia in the final stages of their illness; others show brain disorders even early in the disease. Because the disease is long lasting and highly demoralizing, palliative care in its later stages is necessary, yet it scarcely exists in this country.

Elsewhere in this book we estimate that there are some 30,000 HIV-infected persons in Canada at present. Yet although this number is certain to grow, there is not one institution that sponsors a comprehensive AIDS ambulatory-care program in the entire country.

Some preliminary action has begun: a number of provincial governments have decided to look into remedial action. Ontario has undertaken a study of the needs of hospitals and other organizations to cope with the epidemic, while Quebec has appointed a group of specialists to recommend policies for its prevention, treatment and control.

What the Royal Society proposes
The Committee on AIDS of the Royal Society of Canada took advantage of the greater experience of hospitals in New York and San Francisco in dealing with AIDS, and has made a number of recommendations based on this.

Most important, says the Royal Society report: *"Ad hoc* care of those infected with HIV in Canada must end. AIDS care teams should be set up as quickly as practicable. Focussing patient care in this way is the

most humane, efficient and cost-effective process for AIDS treatment.''
The benefits from the employment of dedicated teams are great, says the
report. Diagnosis can be more rapid and dependable; duplication of tests
is reduced; treatment can be started earlier; disease complications and
side effects from experimental treatments can be identified earlier; drugs
are more easily available for patients; and resources can be optimally
used.

Two principles should guide the planning of care for HIV-infected
persons, says the Royal Society: First, such care should take place
whenever possible in more populous communities where large, often
university-based hospitals and health-care institutions exist, with their
extensive medical resources such as AIDS specialists and special
equipment. The association with a university is important because it
fosters more rapid application of research to practical problems.
Second, it is more compassionate to care for AIDS patients as much as
possible in the community — at home or in extended-care facilities. It
is also considerably less costly; at an average home-care daily cost of
$36-$75, per diem savings could be between $485 and $831 compared
with care in hospitals such as Toronto General. The psychological
benefits of having patients spend their last days in their own
surroundings are simply immeasurable.

The Society makes a number of proposals for patient care in both
large and small centres. One, for a large centre, requires a dedicated
AIDS ward and another dispersing AIDS patients in several wards. In
both cases a multi-disciplinary medical team would serve these patients.
Nurses, social workers and clergy would also be involved both for in-
patients and in an outpatient clinic. Screening and counselling clinics
would be available, which would be staffed by at least a physician and
a social worker. Such clinics would be open at times convenient to
would-be users, and their existence would be made known to public-
health units, private practitioners, gay organizations and others. They
should be inconspicuous, so as not to frighten off those who might want
to visit them, and should not be intimidating for those who do. Central
to the plan is an AIDS centre for co-ordination of and liaison with all the
various elements, which in most cases would be under the aegis of a
university. Community-care agencies would be an integral part of the
scheme.

The system of care recommended for smaller cities differs only in
scale from that proposed for large ones. In smaller centres, for example,

the principal responsibility for the care of HIV patients might fall on a single physician rather than on a multi-disciplinary team. The AIDS centre may not be feasible — or essential — in small cities, however, and its function may be fulfilled by social workers in hospitals and community agencies.

The urgency of implementing these plans needs to be underlined. If Canadians delay in doing so, current problems will become acute, and the level of care now provided for HIV-infected persons, already far from adequate, will deteriorate further. As this happens, the problems will become more and more complex and costly, and the human suffering involved will continue to grow.

Needed: more provincial initiatives

The key role in providing health care for HIV-infected persons and those with AIDS will have to be played by provincial governments because in Canada, health is a provincial responsibility. Provincial governments will, moreover, have to undertake certain initiatives. So far, the bulk of the funds for hospital and educational services for AIDS has come from provincial governments, but a more enterprising approach must be adopted. As it is now, the provinces are *reacting* to requests from those involved in education and treatment of people with HIV or AIDS — waiting for requests for funds for specific purposes and then responding. This approach, the traditional one in the medical and health-care field, is too slow for the emergency situation in which we find ourselves. The provinces must take the initiative and make specific proposals to hospitals, particularly smaller ones.

One urgent need is data gathering for clinical trials of new treatments for AIDS. At present this is handled on a piecemeal basis by hospitals throughout the country, with each hospital being responsible for its own records. Most smaller centres will not have the staff and facilities necessary to manage the increasing amounts of data. Nor is there any way at present to co-ordinate and maintain such data from all these centres across the country. Yet without this co-ordination, it is impossible to conduct properly controlled clinical trials.

Even if this problem can be solved, where will the manpower come from to set up, carry out and evaluate these clinical trials? And how will new drugs be released and distributed on an emergency basis? We have no answers at present.

Patient handling is another problem. The number of persons with

HIV infection and AIDS is fast increasing — and, as we saw in Chapter One, will continue to increase. To take one example, the Ottawa General Hospital at time of writing had about 50 hemophiliac HIV-infected patients and another 200 patients who were HIV-carriers. The latter group was growing by an average of one new patient a week. Medical needs could be handled with current hospital staff, but the hospital had no social-services staff for these patients. Yet for HIV and AIDS patients, such staff is as important as are medical personnel; AIDS patients must be kept track of closely, sometimes for years, the way a general practitioner follows his patients, knowing all about their backgrounds and problems and personalities. Moreover, many AIDS patients have intense social problems, for which social workers are required.

In Quebec, tremendous pressure is being placed on hospitals, particularly in Montreal and particularly in outpatient departments. Facilities have not been developed to handle these pressures, and as Dr. Norbert Gilmore of Montreal's Royal Victoria Hospital said, "We are approaching a crisis." Dr. Gilmore, who is also chairman of the National Advisory Committee on AIDS, said the additional pressures created by AIDS will hasten this crisis because, while the number of AIDS patients is still small, they require comparatively large amounts of care. The pressures are particularly affecting the medical staff who work with AIDS patients; they are simply overworked.

Volunteer efforts

A great deal is owed to community-based volunteer AIDS groups, which began as a result of the gay communities' attempts to meet the needs of its members. In Canada, there are groups based in the major centres of every province except Prince Edward Island, their size varying with the size of the problem. Toronto has about 250 volunteers and a $650,000 budget for 1987/88, while Newfoundland, with few AIDS/HIV cases, has only about 12 volunteers and a budget of less than $1,000. Twenty-five such groups have banded together to form the National AIDS Society.

These groups have developed educational programs not just for gays but for the general population, and have become the major support system for anyone directly affected by the disease. They make referrals to specialists, help with counselling, hold monthly meetings and provide many other services. Canada's first hospice for AIDS patients, which opened in Toronto on March 1, 1988, was set up as a result of the efforts of a community group led by writer June Callwood. Funds and furnishings came from both private and provincial government sources, with operating funds being supplied by the provincial government through St. Michael's Hospital. Called Casey House, after Callwood's son who died in a motorcycle accident, it provides a comfortable refuge for 12 AIDS patients in the last days of their disease.

Volunteer group members donate thousands of hours to such work. Funding arrangements vary, with some groups relying entirely on private donations and others also receiving money from all levels of government and the United Way. An estimate of the value of the services provided free by these groups in 1987 is $2,075,500. Volunteer groups represent an important part of the fight against the spread of AIDS and need continued and increased support.

***

The cost estimates we have presented are just that — estimates based on available data, which at best is scanty. No one knows exactly how much the AIDS epidemic has so far cost Canadians, or exactly how much it will cost in the future. That will depend on many things — advances in treatment, development of a vaccine, even the possibility, remote as it may be, of finding a cure.

Of one thing we can be certain: the costs will be high. To prevent them becoming astronomical, and hindering our progress as a country, we must contain the epidemic and prevent further spread. The best hope for doing this is dealt with in the next chapter.

CHAPTER SIX

What Can Be Done?

In the absence of either a vaccine or a cure for AIDS, we have only one hope of containing the epidemic: education. Everyone must know how AIDS is caused and what to do to prevent becoming HIV-infected. What is more important — we must all *act on* our knowledge.

It has become clear that knowledge does not always equal action. At a press conference following what was called a global summit meeting on AIDS in London, England, in February, 1988, Canada's Minister of Health, Jake Epp, said:

"If you ask Canadians if they are aware of AIDS, there is a very high knowledge base. But the level of knowledge does not change the behavior of high-risk groups, and we so far have limited evidence of how much change in high-risk groups has taken place. There is some, but in many cases knowledge does not translate into action."

What is needed, then, are ways of ensuring not only that the knowledge is there, but that it does become translated into action.

What has been done

Much has already been done to spread the word about AIDS. At least $40 million has already been spent by various governments, and an additional $25-million expenditure was planned for 1987-88. The federal government gives the Canadian Public Health Association alone $800,000 a year for AIDS education and will give community-based groups $1 million a year over the next five years to promote their education programs.

Most provincial governments have set aside money for AIDS-education programs, the amounts being greater in provinces where the numbers of persons with AIDS is greater. For example:

• In British Columbia, provincial and municipal governments share the responsibility, with the latter alone funding community groups. In 1987-88, the provincial government allotted $1.4 million for general education and $5 million for education in schools. The Vancouver Health Department also set aside a portion of its $1-million AIDS budget for education. More money has also gone to HIV-related activities, primarily via a $150,000 grant to AIDS Vancouver.

• Alberta made AIDS education part of the school curriculum, the content being the responsibility of individual school boards. The provincial government funds education for the public through community-based groups.

• Ontario plans to spend $12.5 million over the next five years on AIDS education, with $800,000 to community groups, $6 million to public-health units, $1.2 million to video productions, $700,000 to operate provincial hotlines, $3 million to education and information services and an AIDS office, and $800,000 for the Ontario Public Education Panel on AIDS. Since 1985, the provincial government has given the AIDS committee of Toronto $309,000 to support its education activities. The City of Toronto has set aside $2,546,000 for education from September, 1987, to December, 1989, and $566,000 a year to community groups over the same period.

• Quebec has allotted $800,000 for 1987-88 for AIDS education. A provincial task force with committees on health care, sociolegal, ethical, prevention and research, has been formed and will assess education funding.

• The Northwest Territories has an exemplary AIDS program, in conjunction with Health and Welfare Canada, preparing material for native peoples in 10 languages. The estimated cost is $500,000 in 1987-88, to be shared between the two governments, with the territorial government to become solely responsible in future. Radio and TV messages and pamphlets are available, and visits are made to regional centres where health officials meet with representatives of remote communities.

• Newfoundland and Labrador have not allocated special funds to AIDS education; it is provided through the Public Health Branch. A multimedia campaign began in Autumn, 1987.

• In the Yukon, AIDS expenditures are part of those spent on public health, and interest has been shown in developing a program similar to that of the NWT.

What do surveys tell us?

Despite the spending of all this money, survey results do not seem to unequivocally bear out Health Minister Epps's, remarks about a "high knowledge base" concerning AIDS among Canadians. For example, a survey by Environics Research, carried out in late May and early June, 1987, showed that 87 percent of Canadians believed that HIV can be transmitted through heterosexual intercourse (correct), but a further 15 percent believed that it was possible to get AIDS by using a public washroom (incorrect) and 27 percent thought it was passed through kissing (highly unlikely, and only possible if open sores are present in the mouth). Although the proportion of those answering correctly about heterosexual intercourse (87 percent) is extremely high, can it be concluded that 13 percent did *not* know the correct answer? Not necessarily. The question asked was, "As far as you know, which of the statements on this card describe possible ways that someone can get AIDS" and the respondent was to circle the number beside the following: kissing, touching a person with AIDS, being near a person with AIDS, homosexual sex, heterosexual sex, blood transfusion, public washrooms. There was also a box containing the response Other (specify) and Don't Know or No Answer. Such oversimplified questions do not always draw meaningful answers. After all, it *is* possible to get AIDS in a public washroom — by having unprotected anal sex there with an HIV-infected individual!

Nor do all surveys tell the same story. Another one carried out among 1,507 adults between November 26 and December 4, 1987, by Southam News-Angus Reid, showed that eight of 10 respondents fear getting AIDS from a blood transfusion. This risk, as we have seen earlier, certainly exists, but is infinitesimal compared to many other risks of daily life. Furthermore, almost half those polled worried about getting AIDS from food prepared or served by someone with AIDS, or by visiting a doctor or dentist who has treated an AIDS patient (both of which have never been known to happen). One-third of this sample further believed that they could get AIDS from a swimming pool (impossible if we're talking about being infected simply by using the same pool along with an HIV-infected person).

Such surveys raise questions; for example: how much knowledge is being imparted by current education programs, to what proportion of the population, and with what behavioural-changing effects? And the answer is, we simply don't know (although in the Southam News-Angus Reid poll, while 86 percent believed AIDS could affect all Canadians, only 14 percent said they had changed their behaviour as a result of the AIDS risk).

Some U.S. studies give little reason for complacency about behaviour change. Charles Turner, study director of the Committee on the AIDS Research and the Behavioral and Social Sciences of the National Academy of Sciences, told the AAAS symposium that figures on teenagers and sex showed that those with nine or more sexual partners rated their risk of getting AIDS in the lowest category. Furthermore, many of these did not use condoms. Beth E. Schneider, associate professor of sociology at the University of California, Santa Barbara, said at the same meeting: "There is no evidence I can find to show changes in dating practices, changes in sex practices or in abstinence."

What can we expect from education?
A further question is, how successful can we reasonably expect such programs to be? Is it reasonable to expect, first, that all those who are reached will comprehend everything they are being told and, second, that they will change behaviour appropriately through knowing it? Such questions need researching because we are already aware that there are many areas in which knowing about dangers does not always result in changes in behaviour. The risks of smoking, for example, are well-known, as are those of driving without seat belts, yet many continue to do both. School teachers and parents can tell us, too, that simply providing students or offspring with information does not necessarily lead to prudent behaviour.

One educational difficulty may lie in the feeling of "immortality" that many young people experience — the conviction that death comes only to other people, mostly older ones, and could not possibly touch them. Such an attitude seemed to underly the recent report on a Canadian Broadcasting Corporation newscast that 55 percent of Olympic athletes taking part in a poll said they would knowingly take a drug that could kill them in five years if they thought it would help them to win. To anyone who could make such a statement, death can have no reality.

There seems to be some evidence from the U.S. that AIDS education programs *can* be successful in leading to behavioural change. In San Francisco, a significant decline in unprotected sex has been reported among homosexuals. But how much was this a result of formal education programs and how much simply a result of the fear engendered by seeing their close friends die? Finding the answer may seem an academic exercise, but it matters because of what it tells us about how behavioural change is brought about. Learning this may help in formulating education programs, and effective programs are urgently needed.

We need to examine not just how AIDS education is being attempted but also how our laws may affect AIDS education programs. AIDS has ushered new considerations into a society that as recently as 1969 made it illegal to advertise or encourage the use of contraceptives. For example, the proposed Bill C-54 concerning pornography, if enacted as now worded, could be interpreted in a way that would make it difficult to provide the explicit information necessary to educate people about safer sex practices.

In assessing the adequacy of current AIDS education programs, we must first identify those who still need to know more about the disease and its prevention, determine what they need to know and decide how best to encourage them to want to know. Then we must decide how best to make such information comprehensible and easily retained by these people. Finally, our education efforts need to be evaluated.

Eroticizing the condom

In dealing with AIDS, we must remember that we are dealing with highly pleasurable, private activities and that it is harder to change such behaviour than many other kinds. A moralistic approach will not be useful, in fact it may be counter-productive (60 percent of those polled by Angus Reid, and particularly those aged 18-34, favoured getting safe sex information over moral lectures about promiscuity). What we need to do is try to reduce the risk of infection, not try to change the nature of sexual expression of entire groups of people or wipe out intravenous drug use. The latter is not the purpose of AIDS education and, anyway, experience shows that it will probably fail.

Some researchers propose that, because of the pleasurable and rewarding nature of some of the activities that need to be changed, the behaviours we try to put in their place must also be pleasurable. In practice this means that other rituals must be developed to substitute for needle-sharing rituals among intravenous drug users, and that the use of condoms must be eroticized. The story is told of a prostitute who succeeded in persuading clients to wear condoms by telling them that she found sex more pleasurable that way. In a more general way, condoms could become fashionable among sexually active young people — or even socially de rigueur. One condom manufacturer advertised in *Playboy* magazine with a picture of an attractive young woman saying determinedly: "No Ramses — no sex. I mean it."

Learning from others

Canada may be able to learn from the experience of Australia, where a major public-education campaign has been carried out. Our programs will have to be suited to our people, but theirs can be instructive. Australia's National Advisory Committee on AIDS showed that most Australians had "partial knowledge about AIDS. The small proportion of the sample getting each question wrong were not a small group of people totally lacking in knowledge, but a large group of people partially lacking in knowledge. *People were as confident of their incorrect knowledge as they were of their correct knowledge.*"

The evaluation of the Australian campaign revealed eight barriers to information absorption and behaviour change:

- Prejudice, which results in stereotyping.
- Moral views (a higher level of prejudice was found among frequent churchgoers).
- Blind trust of a partner.
- A belief that AIDS is relevant only to "other people."
- A message that is too reassuring.
- Paranoia, which results from too little reassurance.
- A negative image of condoms.
- The perception that condom use might be seen as an acknowledgement of "guilt."

The Australian AIDS committee also concluded that purely creating awareness or conveying information was unlikely to lead to behaviour changes, and that "a catalyst appears to be needed in many instances to provide a receptive environment for absorption of information." Factors found to be related to behaviour change were relevance, immediacy, fear, knowledge, peer-group pressure and pressure from a sexual partner. The effect of these varied with the individual, and while relevance was considered critical, the problem was that sometimes "the more relevant a piece of communication was, the more it hit a nerve and defensive mechanisms were activated . . . . ''

The San Francisco AIDS Foundation suggests that a person must hold five beliefs in order to change his or her sexual behaviour in relation to AIDS, and that these beliefs can be directly influenced by educational and motivational programs. The beliefs, which tend to occur sequentially, are:

1. That AIDS is a personal threat.
2. That AIDS is preventable and that certain actions will reduce or eliminate risk.
3. That a person is capable of managing these new low-risk behaviours.
4. That sexual satisfaction is still possible while carrying out these new behaviours.
5. That the person's peers will support this new behaviour.

The United Kingdom has also launched a massive educational campaign; leaflets were delivered to every household and all media were used. An evaluation deemed it successful in increasing the general knowledge about HIV, and, perhaps as a result, the evaluation found an increase in sympathy and tolerance for those infected. U.S. research indicates that there is a high correlation between the possession of accurate information and tolerant attitudes. For example, Americans who believe that HIV is transmitted by sneezing are more than twice as likely, as those who do not believe it, to wish to exclude infected students from schools.

Targeting educational programs
Evidence is accumulating that the emphasis in AIDS education programs should be on how people *cannot* get AIDS, rather than how they can. It should stress, for example, that HIV cannot be transmitted through the treated water found in swimming pools, or to blood donors through Red Cross equipment (which is sterilized). It should point out that the risk of receiving HIV-infected blood through a transfusion is less than one in a million, and that if an individual wishes, he or she can avoid even that tiny risk through autologous transfusion. And so on.

Educational programs, furthermore, must be targeted to specific groups of people. They should begin by finding out what such groups already know and feel about AIDS. The perceptions and concerns of different groups will be different. For example, older people, who are more likely to be less sexually active and to be involved in a monogamous relationship, will on the whole have different concerns than the young. People who live in Montreal, Toronto or Vancouver, where the chance of meeting someone with AIDS is much higher than it is in Manitoba or Saskatchewan, may view the question of isolation of people with AIDS differently from those who live in the latter provinces.

IV users and prisoners

Special steps should be taken for groups such as intravenous drug users and prisoners. At present the problem of IV drug users seems less acute here than in the United States, but we do not have much knowledge of this group. Prudence dictates that clean syringes and needles should be made available to prevent the problem of HIV infection from this source from growing. Similarly, education programs for prisoners must recognize the distinctive problems that arise in prisons: these include IV drug use and homosexual sexual encounters (the latter sometimes forced on inmates). Those who run prisons are inhibited from recognizing this fact because such things are not supposed to occur, but they do occur. Under the circumstances, surely it is preferable to make the spread of HIV infection less likely by making condoms and facilities for cleaning needles and syringes available to prisoners, than to continue, ostrich-like, to ignore them.

Educating physicians

Physicians and other health-care providers have as great a need for education programs directed at their requirements as do any other groups. As noted earlier, some tend to avoid dealing with HIV-infected people; this attitude must be discouraged. Education programs for health-care providers should help them to adopt positive attitudes to such patients and help them to treat the patients effectively. Many patients who are uninfected will seek advice from their doctors; physicians must be well-informed to deal with these requests. They will have to know what kind of counsel to offer patients with backgrounds as widely differing, for example, as those of 60-year-olds on the Prairies and 20-year-olds in Montreal; of IV drug users and priests; of children and young adults; of nurses and prostitutes; of immigrants from the Far

East and residents of Rosedale; or of Roman Catholics and fundamentalists. Medical schools and physicians' professional associations will both have parts to play in achieving these goals. In addition, hospitals and other health-care institutions will need to see that their staff training programs are effective — *and* that any special procedures put in place are actually carried out in practice by all staff.

Dealing with AIDS patients can cause many problems for physicians and other hospital staff that are outside their normal experience. Virtually all AIDS patients will enter hospital in the later stages of their disease. Most, being relatively young, will not be prepared to face the prospect of an early death, and because many factors such as cultural background and age may separate them from those who take care of them, hospital staff could also find the situation difficult.

There may, for example, be reluctance to discuss the patient's wishes about death, or if patients have not given directives in advance, house staff may find themselves forced to make decisions about life support and cardiac resuscitation on the spot. Patients may become confused or mentally incompetent at the very time that calls for ethically difficult choices in this regard. And the situation may be complicated by the absence of family members, who normally step in at such times, and the presence of friends or lovers who wish to take the family's place. If the friends or lovers are rejected by the family the situation could be that much worse.

Further problems can be raised by decisions that need to be made about administering treatments that could hasten death. Both the Canadian Law Reform Commission and the Canadian Pediatric Society deem it justifiable to administer drugs to control pain, even if these reduce life expectancy or hasten death. This may leave unresolved the ethical distinction between killing the pain and killing the patient. Questions such as this have led to calls for the legalization of voluntary euthanasia — the deliberate, painless termination of a patient's life at his or her request or with consent, motivated by compassion.

In today's world there is no need for such legalization because of the existence of modern methods of palliative care; with palliative care patients whose condition further medical treatment would not improve, the decision is made to cease such treatment but continue to allay pain and discomfort to the greatest degree possible. Nevertheless, situations sometimes may arise that seem to fall outside all existing rules in caring for the terminally ill. Such situations could cause great anxiety among physicians and other health-care workers, and the whole subject should be dealt with as part of their training.

Telling students about AIDS

Education authorities across the country have already had to grapple with the problem of educating students about the disease. The Canadian Public Health Association commissioned a report that provides an overview of education for Canadian youth in AIDS and other sexually transmitted diseases (STDs). It found that educational authorities in all provinces had moved to develop programs for both junior and senior high school curriculums for 1987/88. It also found that a great deal of material in both print and audio-visual media was already available to schools. Much of it, however, was unsuitable because it was outdated, oriented to the United States, too general, in conflict with community standards, flawed as a teaching tool or considered sexist. The educators were unanimous that AIDS/STD prevention should be taught within the context of human sexuality, which itself should be presented within the context of how students can make responsible choices in life. The report proposed that the CPHA try to get information materials updated and distributed, and that it produce integrated print and video materials appropriate for use in senior high school.

To carry out educational programs in schools effectively, obviously the teachers themselves and those involved in designing the program will have to be sufficiently knowledgeable. How best to ensure this is perhaps a job for teachers' professional associations and such organizations as the Ontario Institute for Studies in Education.

Religious organizations and AIDS

Churches and other religious organizations have a crucial role to play, not only in the education of their adherents but also in helping to set the moral tone of Canadian society. Because AIDS questions are fraught with ethical and moral values, it is vital that the attitudes of religious institutions to AIDS and AIDS patients be carefully considered. Some such institutions might find the subject difficult and even painful to deal with. Others, because of already well-defined attitudes to such aspects as homosexuality, might be tempted to adopt facile attitudes that would tend to polarize public opinion. They would be wise to consider the larger ramifications of their views on society as a whole before adopting what could be a highly divisive stance.

In considering AIDS education, it is instructive once again to look to the past. What must be avoided are the results of the venereal-disease educational campaign launched between 1919 and 1939 in Canada, and described by Jay Cassel in *The Secret Plague*:

> Events during the First World War brought VD to public attention; but while the war shattered the silence on the subject, a major change in attitudes did not follow. Venereal disease did not lose its stigma. In 1930 it could still be reported that those who suffered from VD desired 'to conceal their ailment and avoid the consequent hushed ridicule and criticism of society.' This is a severe judgment on the impact of the education program. By keeping the emphasis on individual conduct, educators maintained the damning implications of venereal infection. VD continued to be associated with wayward conduct, irresponsibility, and infidelity, and with infertility and death. In this way the education program made venereal disease public only to drive it back into secrecy.

CHAPTER SEVEN

The Future

Throughout this book an attempt has been made to put AIDS in perspective, and to deal with its implications for Canadians in a realistic way. This has been done in the belief that it is essential to search for solutions to the problems AIDS poses in a cool-headed, rational way, rather than out of fear. Only in this manner will Canadians be able to deal with the epidemic in their traditional compassionate and humane way.

But this approach must not, in any way, encourage complacency or minimize the seriousness of the situation. We must face the fact that we are confronted by a disease of unprecedented complexity — one that baffles the best brains of science and for which no adequate treatment is remotely in sight. And while the numbers of its victims remain small compared with some of the major killers in modern life, they are still substantial. Furthermore, barring miracles, the fate of those unfortunate individuals has already been sealed.

Elsewhere in this book it has been estimated that between 10,000 and 50,000 Canadians — most probably 30,000 — already are infected by the AIDS virus (an estimate admittedly based on inadequate data, yet one that could as easily turn out to be conservative as exaggerated). Experience indicates that probably all HIV-infected persons will sooner or later show evidence of full-blown AIDS, and that virtually all of these will die from the disease. That means that some 30,000 Canadians will die as a result of this infection within the next several years. And that number could become very much greater if many thousands of Canadians do not change what has been referred to as high-risk behaviour. It helps to put these figures in perspective if we consider that 40,000 Canadian servicemen died *in the whole of the Second World War!*

Put another way, while AIDS ranked only 10th compared to other causes of death for males aged 25-44 in Canada in 1985, by the following year it had moved up into fourth place. And if current epidemiological trends remain constant, male deaths from AIDS in this age group could surpass those from coronary heart disease and become the leading cause of death by 1992.

An attempt has been made to estimate the cost of this catastrophe in terms of money, a task fraught with uncertainty because of the multitude of complications involved, only some of which have been mentioned. Measuring the *human* and *social* cost is impossible — it can only be imagined.

Entering the "AIDS Era"

Some ways have been mentioned in which the challenge of AIDS can be dealt with. Others will be proposed in this chapter and in the recommendations at the end of the book. But what must be stressed is that these consist only of a first tentative groping towards solutions — the beginnings of a process that will extend over many years. We are, as a nation, going to have to learn to live with AIDS for a very long time, perhaps indefinitely. There will be *no* short-term or final solutions. We have to realize that we have entered what may be described as "the AIDS era." The disease we are dealing with has more in common with cancer than with infectious disease such as pneumonia or polio, although in fact no real precedent exists that will help us to cope with it. If we wish to be realistic about the possibilities of development of cures or vaccines for AIDS, we should consider how long medical scientists have been searching for these for cancer, and with what success. The problems are of the same order.

The social problems are equally difficult. In the August, 1987, U.S. National Health Interview Survey, nine out of ten Americans viewed their own risk of getting AIDS as low or non-existent. Yet Americans are much more at risk than Canadians: a million of them are estimated to be HIV-infected. Commenting on this lack of concern, Dr. Harvey V. Fineberg, dean of the Harvard School of Public Health, noted in *Science:*

"Lacking perceived vulnerability, a person is unlikely to change customary habits and behaviors, especially ones that are biologically driven . . . . If there is to be a widespread and persistent shift in behavior related to sex and drugs, it must be grounded in a shift in social norms. Is it imaginable that one day an unmarried couple will find unthinkable the prospect of sexual relations without a condom? That every homosexual couple will practice exclusively safer sex? That every intravenous drug user who cannot quit will incorporate needle cleaning procedures into the ritual of drug use?

"The honest answer to such questions must be: not soon and only with a sustained struggle, if at all. To the strict moralist, these are not even the right questions because they concede unacceptable activities — sexual relations outside of marriage, homosexuality, and illicit drug use."

What, then, are Canada's priorities? First, to stop the spread of HIV. We have discussed ways of doing this in earlier chapters, as well as ways that seem inappropriate. Second, to care for those already ill. Ways of doing this, too, have been discussed. Third — and at this stage of the epidemic this is most important — we must avoid setting harmful precedents on the basis of our present incomplete knowledge and thus tying ourselves down to what might turn out to be inappropriate responses. This is the reason we have stressed the importance of *not* passing laws in haste, particularly those involving HIV testing. The fourth priority, on which in a sense all the rest are based, is to carry out the research necessary to do all the above.

Without research, we will not know how widespread the disease is, and we will not understand how best to contain it. Without research, we will not know how adequately to care for AIDS patients, and we will be unable to find a vaccine or a cure (if indeed such is possible). And without research we will never learn how best to cope with AIDS in a psychological and social sense.

How research should be done
Canada's current research efforts are not nearly commensurate with the size of the health problem AIDS presents to Canadians. In the total number of reported AIDS cases, Canada ranks fourth highest among all countries. Relative to population, we rank 14th highest. In March, 1987, the Panos Institute, an international and policy studies institute, in association with the Norwegian Red Cross, said in *AIDS and the Third World:* "Government response to the AIDS issue [in Canada] has been low key, with education being carried out mainly by gay organizations and the media."

The educational picture has changed since 1987, but we still lag behind such countries as Belgium, Sweden and Switzerland in our research efforts, and these are countries with fewer resources. At least part of the problem is that Canada lacks trained and competent retrovirologists, epidemiologists and immunologists.

Apart from funds allocated for public-health measures, education and prevention programs, AIDS research projects have received only about $8.86 million over the past two years. And while there are at least 85 private or governmental funding agencies, of which 28 seem to have sufficiently broad mandates to be involved in AIDS research, only 14 agencies have in fact supported it. The amount spent by all agencies in 1987-88 on AIDS and HIV research actually *dropped* by $410,000 (to $4.22 million from $4.63 million in 1986-87). Nine percent of this amount was contributed by provincial agencies. During the same year (1987-88), the total spent on education and prevention programs was $24.97 million.

Four federal agencies funded AIDS research between 1986 and 1988. The Medical Research Council (MRC) and the National Health Research and Development Program (NHRDP) of Health and Welfare Canada contributed most, and currently the majority of federal funds go through NHRDP. In addition, in 1986 more than $39 million was promised over five years by the federal government for a major AIDS initiative. Most of this ($22.5 million) was allocated to NHRDP. Two other federally funded agencies, the International Development Research Centre (IDRC) and the Social Sciences and Humanities Research Council (SSHRC), contributed to AIDS research in 1987-88 for the first time. And the Natural Sciences and Engineering Research Council (NSERC), while not directly involved in AIDS research, might contribute through its immunology and virology projects.

Private agencies have also contributed to AIDS research: the British Columbia Medical Services Foundation, the J.P. Bickell Foundation and the National Cancer Institute together have contributed about three percent of the total spent in Canada between 1986 and 1988. And they have supported more than half the training fellowships for AIDS and HIV-related research.

A new approach to AIDS research
The Royal Society Committee on AIDS proposes that, because of the urgency of the problem, and because traditional methods of funding

medical research cannot react quickly and aggressively enough, major new initiatives be undertaken. These would involve new funds and a new national research committee set up to co-ordinate the efforts of the traditional funding bodies (the MRC, SSHRC and NHRDP).

In the traditional method of funding research in Canada, these agencies respond to requests for funds from investigators, who set their own goals. The funding agencies' decisions are based on what is known as "peer review": recommendations for or against the investigators' requests by panels of experts who are the investigators' peers. The new proposal would not simply be *responsive,* as this method is; instead it would adopt an *active* role in working with investigators. It might, for example, develop research contracts, expedite interactions between investigators in different parts of the country, promote conferences and perhaps even provide advice to investigators whose proposals fall short of the demands of peer review. The goal would be actively to help in getting more research in AIDS going.

In addition to this new national committee, new AIDS committees would be set up by each of the traditional funding bodies to work with the national committee. Moreover, since there is no major centre in Canada where individual scientists can pool their talents in AIDS research, two or three groups of scientists would be established to allow some of the best investigators in the country to develop special research programs. And because of the shortage of Canadian scientists in appropriate fields of research, some will have to be invited from abroad. This will call for special exemptions from current immigration policy.

All these initiatives will, of course, cost money. The Royal Society Committee on AIDS has estimated that the total will be about $35 million a year for research in biomedicine, epidemiology, economics and public health, and for training programs for scientists and operating grants.

What can ordinary Canadians do?
Dr. Norbert Gilmore, chairman of the National Advisory Committee on AIDS, likes to tell people that what Canadians need most in the face of the AIDS epidemic is courage. "We need courage," he says, "to face the disease and to learn how to cope with it."

This means looking at the facts and their implications squarely and coolly. Fear is not the best basis on which to make decisions — but fear of dangerous consequences can sometimes become a healthy stimulus to prudent behaviour. Fear is only dangerous when it leads to unreasoning reactions, when it becomes panic.

Unreasoning fear, or panic, is at least partly behind such actions as the burning down of the house in which HIV-infected children lived in Arcadia, Florida, in 1987, an action that produced a widespread feeling of revulsion. It is this sort of action we in Canada will want to guard against. Commenting on it, James Merriam, a reporter for United Press International, said at a meeting of the Radio and Television News Directors Association:

"One of the questions people ask me all the time is: Isn't there too much media coverage of AIDS? I'm a good example of what media coverage can do, because I wrote a lot of early AIDS stories and noticed the symptoms. My doctor had never tested anybody for AIDS before. I said, 'I've got the symptoms, and we need to test me for it.' I ended up getting treatment and am probably alive today because of that.

"I also think Arcadia, Florida, last week shows that there's a long way to go towards educating people, and the major way that's going to happen is through the mass media.

"It's not going to take one series. Or one week. Or one month. But hammering it in time after time. Story after story. Until there's some understanding. Unfortunately, the other thing that will help bring people around is that more and more people will get to know somebody who has AIDS. And that's going to help change attitudes."

Participating in the same discussion, which was organized by the Media Resource Service of the Scientists' Institute for Public Information, Laurie Garrett, science correspondent for National Public Radio, said about media coverage of AIDS:

"There are a couple of other things you might want to consider. One is a tendency to emphasize the AIDS story from the perspective of human behaviour: How does a community respond when the epidemic comes to town? But even if you do everything possible to present a balanced sense of risk, most people will feel that their fears have been validated by seeing the fears expressed by the individual on camera.

"The only way that you can cut through that is by bringing in the science — the stuff that nobody wants to do on radio and television because it's so hard to do, because you're afraid that the second you start with science, the ratings go down. But if you don't explain what science knows about AIDS, you're doing a serious disservice. If you only show the hysteria, there's a sense that we don't understand it, and everybody is going to be hysterical. One of our jobs is to say it's not that mysterious. A miraculous amount has been discovered in a very short time.''

Those remarks were obviously directed at the media, but they apply in a way to all Canadians. If the media have a responsibility to allay hysteria by presenting the facts, we in the audience have a responsibility to listen and to learn. We can be sure that we will not be alone in doing so. Learning about AIDS and coming to terms with AIDS are tasks that will have to be shared not just by Canadians, but by all the world's peoples, if we are to avert a major global catastrophe.

What Everyone Wants To Know About AIDS

Q. What is AIDS?

A. AIDS (Acquired Immunodeficiency Syndrome) is a disease caused by a virus that attacks the body's immune system, leading to its collapse. This leaves the infected person vulnerable to a number of other infections or cancers. Some of these, though not usually fatal to a person with a normal immune system, become lethal to someone with AIDS.

Q. How does one become infected by the AIDS virus?

A. The AIDS virus is known as HIV (Human Immunodeficiency Virus). If HIV gets into the bloodstream, it infects and destroys white blood cells called T-helper cells. These cells orchestrate the immune system's response to infection, so that when they are destroyed this system cannot function properly. HIV can enter the bloodstream (a) via sexual contact with an infected person, (b) through contaminated needles or syringes used for drug injection, or (c) through transfusion of infected blood or blood products. An infected mother can also transmit the virus to her baby before or during birth, and possibly through breast-feeding. In Canada, the most common means of transmission is (a). Since November, 1985, when the Canadian Red Cross put special precautions into effect, (c) has virtually disappeared as a cause of HIV infection.

Q. Can you get AIDS by associating with people who have the disease?

A. No. The AIDS virus is not spread by casual contact (i.e., shaking hands, from toilet seats, etc.). Those who live in the same quarters as persons with AIDS, or who work with them, are not at risk. AIDS is spread only through sexual contact with an infected person or through transmission of the virus from his or her blood to yours. Nor has there been any case known to result from kissing.

Q. How widespread is AIDS in Canada?

A. Nobody knows for certain because persons infected with HIV may show no symptoms and therefore not realize they have been infected, and because we cannot be sure all AIDS cases have been reported. However, by May, 1988, the Federal Centre for AIDS had received reports of 1,765 cases of AIDS (1,732 adults and 33 children), among which were 984 deaths. The Royal Society of Canada's AIDS study estimates that about 30,000 persons in Canada had been infected with HIV by September, 1987, though the figure could be as low as 10,000 or as high as 50,000.

Q. Where did the AIDS virus come from?

A. Its origin is unknown. Because stored blood from some African countries shows evidence of the virus's presence as far back as 1959, some have speculated that it arose in Africa. But similar studies have not been carried out on blood from Europe or North America, so this evidence is inconclusive. Also, while AIDS-like diseases are now known to have appeared in Africa in the late 1970s, some cases also showed up in the United States around the same time.

Q. Is AIDS always fatal?

A. AIDS is the final stage of the disease caused by HIV infection. It is invariably fatal, usually within two years of its onset. However, a person infected by HIV may show no symptoms for weeks, months or years. Most experts now believe that all those infected will eventually develop AIDS, though it is not known within what period of time in any individual case.

Q. What are the symptoms of AIDS?

A. There may be many, some of which may be those one associates ordinarily with other diseases, including influenza. Only a physician can tell whether the diagnosis is really AIDS. Early symptoms for those in risk groups may include:

• Swollen glands in the neck, below the ears, in the groin or armpits, persisting over more than a month.

• Unexplained weight loss of more than 10 pounds or 10 percent of body weight in two months.

• Persistent fatigue and loss of appetite.

• Fevers and night sweats over a number of days or weeks.

• Persistent diarrhea.

Q. How is HIV infection diagnosed?

A. A diagnosis must be made by a physician with the help of a physical examination, a medical history and blood and/or other tests. Blood tests may include a screening test called ELISA (enzyme-linked immunosorbent assay) and a confirmatory test called the Western Blot. These tests detect antibodies to HIV in the blood. No simple test exists to demonstrate the presence in the body of the virus itself. Nor can any test *by itself* diagnose HIV infection or the presence of AIDS.

Q. Shouldn't everyone be tested so that we would know for sure how many people are infected and who they are?

A. There are many arguments against universal testing, and also against compulsory testing. First, tests alone should not be used for diagnosis, as noted above. In low-risk groups, such as the general population, they may produce false positives (i.e., show an HIV infection where none exists) and false negatives (show no HIV infection where one does, in fact, exist). The latter can occur because it takes some days, weeks or months for the body to produce antibodies after infection has occurred. Second, because of the widespread fear of AIDS, those diagnosed as being HIV-infected are often discriminated against in a variety of ways. And despite attempts to keep the diagnosis confidential, it may leak out. As for making tests compulsory, many of those most likely to be infected would try to avoid them — yet they are the people most in need of assistance in coping with the results of infection.

Q. But shouldn't testing be compulsory for immigrants and visitors to Canada?

A. This, too, would be impractical. First because of cost: Canada has had an average of 90,000 immigrants a year for the past five years and about 65-million visitors. Also, each year thousands of Canadians return from visits to other countries, some of which have a high prevalence of AIDS. The United States, with which we have virtually free traffic in both directions, for example, has about 50,000 recorded cases of AIDS and perhaps a million HIV-infected persons. But as well as being exceedingly costly, testing of visitors would not be feasible administratively. Furthermore, the return would be extremely low in numbers of cases uncovered. Finally, testing on entry would not detect those who had been infected too close to the testing date to show antibodies.

Q. Who are those most likely to become infected?

A. Heterosexuals who have many sexual partners; people who use contaminated drug-injection equipment; and homosexuals with many partners. Those who received blood transfusions or blood products prior to 1985 and persons from countries with a high prevalence of HIV have also been more at risk, as have sexual partners of the above.

Q. How can infection be avoided?

A. By practising "safer sex" habits, by not having sexual intercourse with those in high-risk groups, and by refraining from intravenous drug abuse. If drug injections *are* practised, by making sure that only sterilized needles and syringes are used. Health workers, laboratory personnel, funeral directors and others who work with body fluids should strictly follow safety procedures that have been recommended by federal and provincial authorities to minimize exposure not just to HIV but also to hepatitis B and other blood-borne diseases.

Q. What is "safer sex"?

A. Since HIV is carried by semen, vaginal secretions and other body fluids, it is important to avoid contact with those of a possibly infected person. Any sexual practice that could result in exchange of blood or body fluids with an infected person is risky. Condoms will protect against HIV infection when properly used. The safest sexual behaviour, of course, would be to refrain from sexual intercourse altogether, but this is hardly practical for most people. The next safest is to have sexual intercourse with only one partner who is known not to have been exposed to the AIDS virus. The greater the number of sexual partners one has, the greater one's risk of being infected.

Q. Why not just quarantine everyone who tests positive for the AIDS virus?

A. Quarantine is used for infections spread by casual contact (e.g., sneezing or coughing, contact with household utensils). AIDS is not spread in this way. Quarantine also is used as a temporary measure with diseases that can be treated or cured. There is no effective treatment and no cure for AIDS, so quarantine would amount to lifetime segregation of people with AIDS — a cruel punishment and one subject to abuse because it would be subject to no legal safeguards. Such a punishment would also be ineffective as a disease-control measure because many apparently healthy people may also be infected with HIV without knowing it. Finally, if the estimate of 30,000 HIV-infected persons in Canada is correct, quarantine would be completely impractical.

Q. Should all hospital patients be tested on admission?

A. No: testing is unnecessary. Only about one in 5,000 hospital patients without AIDS symptoms, excluding those already known to be positive, will probably be found to be HIV-infected. The risk to health-care workers from an accidental needle puncture from these patients will be about one in 500,000, and even lower for exposure to infected body fluids in other ways. Furthermore, the results of patients' tests would have to be kept confidential and counselling provided. Both would be extremely difficult to accomplish.

Q. Should testing of teachers and students be mandatory?

A. No, because transmission of the AIDS virus does not occur in the normal school setting. What is needed in schools are adequate education programs showing how to avoid infection.

Q. A recent estimate of the risk of contracting AIDS through a single, unprotected incident of sexual intercourse with an infected person has been put at one in 500. Isn't that low?

A. Not if you consider the consequences of that one chance in 500: a painful disease, possibly severe social and personal consequences and certain early death. It is also instructive to compare this risk with others often taken. For example, you can fly 6,000 miles in a jet and your risk of dying will only increase by one in a million.

Q. Isn't it true that the AIDS virus has not spread as fast as feared among the heterosexual population in North America?

A. Yes, but this is no cause for complacency. The disease *is present* among heterosexuals, and will continue to spread if each individual does not help prevent it. As of May, 1988, 42 people in Canada had died from AIDS contracted through sexual intercourse from partners in risk groups. Those who have sex with *many* partners are at increased risk: whenever they have sex with one new partner they are, in effect, having sex with all those that person has slept with during the past eight years, because it takes that long on average for an AIDS infection to appear.

Q. What are the chances of curing AIDS with some of the new drugs we have read about?

A. Medical experts say that of all the current new drugs available, there
    is no reason to expect that any will provide a cure for AIDS.
    Carefully controlled trials are essential to evaluate all new drugs,
    and there is no point in making widely available drugs that have not
    been properly evaluated.

Recommendations

The following are the recommendations of the Royal Society of Canada's panel of experts in their study, *AIDS: A Perspective for Canadians.*

Prevention of spread

We recommend that the federal government, through its own agencies and with the World Health Organization, take an active and supportive role in combating AIDS worldwide.

We recommend that the three levels of government in Canada cooperate in providing funding for HIV-education programs promoting health. At least $80 million should be allocated to these programs each year. The design and responsibility for carrying out these programs may well involve substantial roles for volunteer community groups.

We recommend expanded and targeted education programs and information about the prevention of HIV transmission, in order to address the specific needs of all sectors of the public.

We recommend that all education programs include an evaluation component to provide continuing assessment and changes if necessary to produce the most effective approach. Concerted efforts also should be made immediately to evaluate the effectiveness of the wide variety of existing educational programs.

We recommend that every workplace develop education programs tailored to the conditions of the workplace and designed cooperatively by management, unions, employees and occupational health and safety representatives.

We recommend that all health-care personnel be trained in appropriate infection control procedures and that such procedures be implemented consistently.

We recommend that condoms be available for inmates in correctional institutions and for others who choose not to refrain from sexual behaviours that could transmit HIV.

We recommend that free condoms, needles, syringes and facilities for decontaminating needles be made available to injection drug users who choose not to refrain from behaviours that could transmit HIV.

We recommend that facilities for decontaminating needles be made readily available to inmates in correctional institutions.

We recommend that HIV-infected women and men be discouraged from having children. Pregnancy may accelerate the course of the mother's disease, and there is a high probability that HIV will be transmitted to the child.

We recommend that provincial professional regulatory legislation provide that, where a health-care provider has reasonable cause to believe that an HIV-infected person is in such mental, physical or emotional condition as to be dangerous to others, and that disclosure of information about the patient is necessary to prevent the threatened danger, the health-care provider may disclose such information to the person or persons in danger without the consent of the patient. Disclosure made under that reasonable belief shall not amount to professional misconduct.

Testing for HIV

We recommend the carefully considered use of voluntary and anonymous testing as an adjunct to education and public health initiatives for controlling further spread of the disease. Such testing should be made available to all Canadians through readily accessible testing clinics that should also provide counselling before and after the test.

We recommend that the finding of a positive result in a screening test for HIV antibodies must always be considered as tentative and that a person must not be reported as seropositive unless the screening test result is validated by one or more confirmatory test.

We recommend that federal and provincial agencies review and institute appropriate regulations to ensure that HIV antibody tests for Canadians are carried out only in approved Canadian laboratories using standardized reagents and methods and having trained, qualified personnel to interpret the results.

We recommend the direct use of blood, organs and tissues, including sperm, ova and bone, only from donors who do not have evidence of HIV infection.

We reject proposals calling for routine mandatory testing of all hospital patients.

We reject proposals calling for mandatory testing of persons seeking permanent residence in Canada.

We reject proposals calling for mandatory testing of students, teachers or other persons employed in schools.

We recommend that reporting laws be amended to provide that the reporting of HIV seropositivity and AIDS should not identify the person.

We recommend that provincial reporting laws be amended to allow anonymous testing for research purposes.

Care and treatment of the infected

We recommend that the federal and provincial governments cooperate in the establishment of a system for the care of those infected with HIV, along the lines of the system proposed in a background paper to this Report.

We recommend that a survey be undertaken immediately on a provincial or regional basis to determine the human and institutional resource requirements for the proposed system of care of those infected with HIV.

We recommend that social benefits be improved to provide adequate financial support for people with AIDS and their dependent families. We further recommend that subsidized housing be made available to those HIV-infected persons who have social or housing problems resulting from their infection.

We recommend that compensation be provided to persons infected with HIV through the transfusion of blood or blood products.

We recommend that all human rights legislation be amended to prohibit discrimination based on evidence of HIV infection, perceived HIV infection, sexual orientation or perceived sexual orientation. We further recommend that policy makers and the general public be educated about such human rights legislation.

We recommend that there be no general isolation or quarantine of HIV-seropositive people or of people with AIDS.

We recommend that the provinces enact legislation imposing liability for breaches of confidentiality without proof of actual damage. Liability should be for a predetermined amount sufficiently large to act as a significant deterrent to such breaches.

We recommend that legislation be enacted to provide compensation for those injured by vaccination or by other preventive and medical programs that may be developed for HIV infection.

Organization of research

Because of the importance of developing a coordinated approach to research funding, we recommend that a meeting of federal and provincial ministers be convened as early as possible to discuss appropriate mechanisms for sharing the responsibility of supporting AIDS-related research.

We recommend the establishment of a federally funded resource group, analogous to the clinical trials group of the National Cancer Institute of Canada, to plan and coordinate both publicly funded and industry-sponsored HIV-related clinical trials.

We recommend that the Social Sciences and Humanities Research Council (SSHRC) establish studies of sexual behaviour to assist in the design of education and public health programs and to establish a database of sexual knowledge, attitudes and practices among Canadians.

We recommend that the Medical Research Council, the Social Science and Humanities Research Council, and the National Health and Research Development Program use proactive dedicated AIDS committees to promote and support HIV-related research in their respective fields.

We recommend that a national research committee be formed to coordinate the AIDS-related research efforts of the Medical Research Council, the Social Science and Humanities Research Council, and the National Health and Research Development Program and perhaps to coordinate other research problems that may transcend their traditional mandates. For example, this committee could be set up under the aegis of the Royal Society of Canada.

We recommend that group programs be established in which personnel with expertise in many different aspects of AIDS-related research can pool their talents to undertake research that is highly cost-effective.

We recommend the development of four multidisciplinary research units that combine the disciplines of clinical epidemiology, public health, economics, and the other social sciences, and the creation of one unit for health policy research.

Areas of research
To replace assumptions with data, we recommend that epidemiological surveys be carried out to estimate the number of HIV-infected persons in Canada.

We recommend anonymous sample surveys, approved by institutional ethics or human experimentation committees, as the preferred avenue for achieving the goal of HIV epidemiologic surveillance.

We recommend clinical and epidemiological studies to determine the relationship of possible cofactors to the susceptibility to infection and to the development of HIV-associated diseases.

We recommend epidemiological surveys to monitor the spread of HIV infection among injection drug users, using voluntary and/or anonymous testing.

We recommend studies on the use and meaning of education in relation to the changing sexual and social behaviour among three sectors of our society: people who are HIV-infected, people who are at risk of becoming HIV-infected, and people who work with these two groups.

We recommend studies on the effectiveness of voluntary agencies in conveying accurate and change-inducing information and support to subgroups engaged in activities within or outside the law, to those who are unable to read or hear, and to those who may not be responsible for their own behaviour such as the mentally handicapped. The scope and methods of funding for such agencies will also have to be determined.

We recommend research to determine the means by which high-risk groups, such as injection drug users and others operating outside the norm or laws of society, may be most effectively contacted and influenced.

We recommend studies of how institutions can best achieve their goals or promopting behavioural change in those members of society who are HIV-infected or who are at risk of becoming HIV-infected. Such institutions include, among others, correctional institutions, educational institutions, and hospitals and other health-care centres.

We recommend cost-analysis and cost-effectiveness studies of selected projects of community support for HIV-infected persons.

We recommend a large multiwave survey of the adult and adolescent Canadian population. This survey would provide currently lacking information about sexual practices, ideas and feelings about AIDS, patterns of social ties and behaviour relevant to the spread of sexual diseases, trust in various sources of information, and other factors bearing on the future spread of HIV-infection and means of prevention. These data will be useful for both network analysis and epidemiological purposes.

We recommend societal and anthropological studies of the relationship between HIV-infected persons and those who interact with them, in order to understand the dynamics of population behaviour, the course of discriminatory behaviour and change, and the basis on which information changes values, attitudes and behaviour.

We recommend a prospective study of newly diagnosed patients from the Montreal, Toronto or Vancouver areas, for a predetermined time, to determine the direct costs of treating HIV infection.

We recommend that clinical trials of preventive and therapeutic measures be administered with full disclosure of foreseeable risks and benefits, informed consent, and approval from an institutional ethics or human experimentation committee. We seriously question the ethics of using volunteers from the military, children, or inmates of custodial institutions.

Clinging to Misconceptions

Some people working in the AIDS field have noticed a curious phenomenon: many members of the public not only hold misconceptions
about the disease, but are loathe to let these false beliefs go.

Dr. Alastair Clayton, director-general of Canada's Federal Centre for
AIDS, says the major misconceptions concern transmission of the AIDS
virus.

"There seems to be an inability to accept transmission routes," he
says. "There is no wish to accept that the routes are through blood and
semen. People always ask if the virus can be spread through food, by
mosquitos, in swimming pools, through touching, from toilet seats and
telephones, and so on. I can stand up at my lectures and tell them this
doesn't happen, but they still ask the same questions at the end of the
lecture."

Dr. Clayton thinks it's part of a "plague mentality" — a pattern of
thought that has occurred repeatedly during the plagues of history. At
first people show a wish to understand how the infection spreads. Then
they misinterpret what they are told. Then they deny the facts. Hysteria
or panic follows, and finally they ostracize those who fall victim to the
disease and perhaps quarantine them.

"It's happened with all past plagues, such as the Black Death in
Europe and smallpox," says Dr. Clayton. "Blame is placed outside
ourselves. Sometimes it's easy to find scapegoats, such as Asians in the
case of smallpox during the first half of the century. People in effect say
to themselves, 'It can't possibly be *my* fault.' So they blame people who
are not like themselves."

Such attitudes create a ready audience for books and media programs
that blame minorities such as homosexuals or conspiracies of various
kinds. A U.S. - originated religious program featuring the evangelist
Jack Van Impe, aired in Canada, that dealt with the AIDS epidemic as
a divinely inspired retribution against homosexuals, is one such

example. Another is a book entitled *The AIDS Cover-up? The Real and Alarming Facts About AIDS.*

"I myself have been accused on radio talk shows of concealing the truth," says Dr. Clayton. "After trying to give the facts, I've been told by callers: 'I don't believe you. You're covering up.' "

The AIDS Cover-up? contains what seems to be a careful selection of quotations and references from highly respected authorities to prove the author's contention that the real truth about AIDS is being concealed from the public. The background and qualifications of the author, Gene Antonio, do not appear in the second edition (1987), published by Ignatius Press, San Francisco, but Dr. Clayton believes he is a sociologist.

Part of the problem with the book, Dr. Clayton believes, is that the author makes partial quotations from experts and then adds his own interpretation of what they mean, sometimes distorting them in the process. The result is sometimes half-truth. Dr Clayton characterized the book (with whose author he appeared — and whom he challenged — on the CBC program "Cross-Country Checkup") as being "well-written, but full of persuasive grammar which tends to lead the readers into making conclusions that are incorrect.

"There is a small vocal minority that is becoming more influential in spreading false ideas about the AIDS epidemic," Dr. Clayton contends.

One misconception about the spread of AIDS is that it is easy to contract the disease. "It is relatively easy to get infected with HIV during anal intercourse if there is a lot of trauma and a lot of blood and if the person doing the penetrating is highly infectious, but it is difficult to get it any other way except through blood transfusions," Dr. Clayton said. "In male-female sexual intercourse, it seems to require an average of more than 100 sexual encounters, unprotected by a condom, before you can pick it up from an infected partner."

Dr. Clayton sees this not as a reason for people to be careless about safer sex strategies, but encouraging. "Safer sex *can* be practised and will reduce the incidence of the disease. Relative to homosexual transmission, heterosexual cases are not increasing and the rate remains between two and three percent of the total number. In Canada, very few females (less than 100) have acquired it. And because of this slow heterosexual spread we are in a position to stop it."

Even among health-care workers exposed to the virus, transmission has so far not been a major problem, Dr. Clayton says. "No health-care worker in Canada who is not in a high-risk category (i.e. homosexual or drug abuser) has become infected as a result of occupational exposure, and there have been only nine in the entire world," he said.

Once again, this is not cause for complacency, though it is reassuring. "AIDS has allowed us to reinforce the precautions we take in dealing with other blood-borne disease."